the**facts**

Diabetes

→ also available in the**facts** series

Eating disorders: the**facts**
FIFTH EDITION
Abraham

Sexually transmitted infections:
the**facts**
SECOND EDITION
Barlow

Thyroid disease: the**facts**
FOURTH EDITION
Vanderpump and Tunbridge

Living with a long-term illness:
the**facts**
Campling

Prenatal tests: the**facts**
DeCrespigny

Obsessive-compulsive disorder:
the**facts**
THIRD EDITION
De Silva

The pill and other forms of
hormonal contraception: the**facts**
SIXTH EDITION
Guillebaud

Myotonic dystrophy: the**facts**
Harper

Ankylosing spondylitis: the**facts**
Khan

Prostate cancer: the**facts**
Mason

Multiple sclerosis: the**facts**
FOURTH EDITION
Matthews

Essential tremor: the**facts**
Plumb

Panic disorder: the**facts**
SECOND EDITION
Rachman

Tourette syndrome: the**facts**
Robertson

ADHD: the**facts**
Selikowitz

Dyslexia and other learning
difficulties: the**facts**
SECOND EDITION
Selikowitz

Schizophrenia: the**facts**
SECOND EDITION
Tsuang

Depression: the**facts**
Wassermann

Polycystic ovary syndrome:
the**facts**
Elsheikh and Murphy

Autism and Asperger syndrome:
the**facts**
Baron-Cohen

Motor neuron disease: the**facts**
Talbot and Marsden

Muscular dystrophy: the**facts**
THIRD EDITION
Emery

Stroke: the**facts**
Lindley

Osteoarthritis: the**facts**
Arden, Arden, and Hunter

Cosmetic surgery: the**facts**
Waterhouse

the**facts**

Diabetes

DAVID MATTHEWS

and the team at the Oxford Centre for
Diabetes, Endocrinology and Metabolism

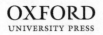

OXFORD
UNIVERSITY PRESS

OXFORD
UNIVERSITY PRESS

Great Clarendon Street, Oxford OX2 6DP

Oxford University Press is a department of the University of Oxford.
It furthers the University's objective of excellence in research, scholarship,
and education by publishing worldwide in

Oxford New York

Auckland Cape Town Dar es Salaam Hong Kong Karachi
Kuala Lumpur Madrid Melbourne Mexico City Nairobi
New Delhi Shanghai Taipei Toronto

With offices in

Argentina Austria Brazil Chile Czech Republic France Greece
Guatemala Hungary Italy Japan Poland Portugal Singapore
South Korea Switzerland Thailand Turkey Ukraine Vietnam

Oxford is a registered trade mark of Oxford University Press
in the UK and in certain other countries

Published in the United States
by Oxford University Press Inc., New York

© Oxford University Press, 2008

The moral rights of the authors have been
Database right Oxford University Press (m

First published 2008

All rights reserved. No part of this publicat
stored in a retrieval system, or transmitted,
without the prior permission in writing of (
or as expressly permitted by law, or under
reprographics rights organization. Enquirie
outside the scope of the above should be se
Oxford University Press, at the address abo

You must not circulate this book in any oth
and you must impose this same condition on any acquirer

British Library Cataloguing in Publication Data

Data available

Library of Congress Cataloging in Publication Data
Diabetes / Matthews [et al.]
   p.cm. — (The facts)
   ISBN-13: 978–0–19–923266–6
1. Diabetes—Popular works. I. Matthews, David, 1947–
   RC660.4.D482 2008
   616.4′62—dc22

                                                            2008004568

ISBN 978–0–19–923266–6

10 9 8 7 6 5 4 3

Typeset in Plantin
by Cepha Imaging Pvt. Ltd., Bangalore, India
Printed in Great Britian by Ashford Colour Press Ltd

Whilst every effort has been made to ensure that the contents of this book are as complete, accurate,
and up-to-date as possible at the date of writing, Oxford University Press is not able to give any
guarantee or assurance that such is the case. Readers are urged to take appropriately qualified
medical advice in all cases. The information in this book is intended to be useful to the general
reader, but should not be used as a means of self-diagnosis or for the prescription of medication.

Foreword

I was diagnosed as diabetic one Saturday morning in 1985. I had walked along to report that I had a constant and unquenchable thirst (no surprise to my GP!), and that I was now looking forward to sweetened fruit-juice—even to iced water—almost as much as to my customary alcoholic beverages. 'Any other symptoms?' Yes, an overwhelming tiredness on returning home from work at about 5.30 p.m., when all I wished for was to get into bed—sometimes even *before* The Archers. My GP checked my blood-sugar level ('Off the scale,' he informed me), and immediately sent me off to hospital for a fortnight, with an ominous, yet accurate, prediction that I would be 'on insulin' for the rest of my life.

One might have thought that thereafter I would soon become au fait with all this diabetic business; and indeed for many years I was regularly asked to air my semi-ignorance in interviews and articles, at conferences, and on radio. Almost invariably did I mention the two sombre options: either diabetes is going to control your life, or you are going to control diabetes. I usually added in a flippant manner that we shouldn't take diabetes all that seriously, and that the only real trouble was carting around all the kit and the medication. I now realize that I could not have been of much help to those foolish enough to listen to me. What examples did I give of my frivolous attitude? Well, blood-sugar readings had never troubled me overmuch; and when appointment times came round, I used to take such readings (unless they were too high!) four or five times on each of the two days prior to the appointment, and then, with devious fabrication, extrapolate these readings backwards for the previous two weeks. I also wish that during those years I had been far more honest with my eminent consultants, although I'm sure that they very soon smelled a whole colony of rats when I invariably answered 'Fine!' to each of their queries concerning weight, blood-pressure, sexual prowess, and alcoholic consumption.

'A little learning is a dangerous thing,' dear readers. And over recent years I have seen the error of my ways, conscious that my own past sins are now finding me out. It was, in my case, diabetes which had the upper hand—not me. So, my message now? Whichever type of diabetes we have, whether its effects upon us are 'mild' or 'severe', everyone of us must take it very seriously indeed. It has taken me (now in my 78th year) an awfully long time to face up to this simple truth, has it not?

So what about this book, *Diabetes: the facts?* Many medical journals and tracts are couched in a quasi-specialist, sesquipedalian obscurity; and my only contribution to the last one I was asked to read was to beg my colleagues (I was on the committee!) to record their findings in such a way as to be readily understood by GPs and above—let alone by laymen and below. Now, blessedly, the hallmarks of this publication are simplicity and lucidity; and I heartily congratulate the writer(s) for knowing what 'good English' is all about. Moreover the layout, diagrams, and illustrations here are so cleverly managed that the study of this handbook becomes a pleasingly valuable refresher-course for all of us. I found the FAQ ('frequently asked questions') boxes of special interest; and (at my age) the first chapter I considered carefully was 'The future', where the various authors have dispensed their wisdom concerning heart attacks, strokes, feet, neuropathy, retinopathy, etc.—the last two splendid words fully explained once more in the extensive glossary.

In short the book is comprehensive and comprehensible; and if we referred to it as *The Definitive Bible for Diabetes*, I am sure that Professor David Matthews would be highly delighted.

Colin Dexter, February 2008

Contents

About the authors

Professor David Matthews MA, DPhil, BM, BCh, FRCP

The Oxford Centre for Diabetes, Endocrinology and Metabolism

David Matthews is currently Professor of Diabetes Medicine, University of Oxford, Consultant Physician, Oxford Radcliffe Hospitals NHS Trust, Chairman of the Oxford Centre for Diabetes, Endocrinology and Metabolism, and he is Medical Tutor at Harris Manchester College, Oxford. He is Co-director of the UK Diabetes Research Network. He divides his time between patient care, research, and teaching.

His academic research interests include mathematical modelling of insulin resistance, homeostatic model assessment of beta-cell function and insulin resistance, ketones, therapeutic agents in type 2 diabetes, global obesity epidemic—Oxford Health Alliance—and he is deputy co-ordinator of the UK Prospective Study of Diabetes (UKPDS). He has authored more than 200 publications and is on the editorial boards of several professional journals.

He has served as Chairman of the Diabetes UK research grants committee and been on the Board of Trustees. He is currently a grant committee member for the European Foundation for the Study of Diabetes (EFSD) and special prize committee member for the European Association for the Study of Diabetes (EASD). He co-ordinates the EASD Robert Turner training course in diabetes.

Sue Beatty

Diabetes research nurse, The Oxford Centre for Diabetes, Endocrinology and Metabolism

Sue Beatty is a clinical research nurse based at the Oxford Centre for Diabetes, Endocrinology and Metabolism. She has worked in diabetes research for 6 years. She has been involved in a wide range of research studies and has a particular interest in islet transplantation.

Pam Dyson

Research dietician, University of Oxford

Pam Dyson has been involved with the nutritional management of diabetes and obesity for over 25 years. She began her working life with the Medical Research Council at the Dunn Nutrition Unit in Cambridge, and since then has practised as a community dietician and diabetes specialist dietician both for in- and outpatients, and has been closely involved with clinical research. Since 2003, she has been employed by Oxford University as a diabetes research dietician and she is involved both with external projects (usually multicentre diabetes trials) and in-house projects (at present various educational programmes and dietary intervention trails for weight loss). The expansion of this role has included registration at Oxford Brookes University for a PhD study evaluating dietary education for people with type 2 diabetes. Her main interests are in the delivery of diabetes dietary education, behavioural aspects of lifestyle change, and weight management.

Laurie King

Podiatrist, The Oxford Centre for Diabetes, Endocrinology and Metabolism

Laurie King has been a clinical podiatrist for the past 28 years in the NHS, the last 24 years specializing in diabetic foot and wound healing.

Dr Niki Meston

Clinical research fellow, The Oxford Centre for Diabetes, Endocrinology and Metabolism

Niki Meston qualified in medicine from Southampton University and moved into the speciality of clinical biochemistry 13 years ago. This involves patient care in metabolic medicine including in the fields of diabetes, endocrinology, lipid, and metabolic bone disease over this time. Her work also involves interpreting results of blood investigations in the clinical biochemistry laboratory, and teaching clinical biochemistry to undergraduate and postgraduate students.

Dr Aparna Pal

Specialist registrar in Diabetes, Endocrinology and General Medicine

Aparna did her undergraduate medical training at Oxford University Medical School and has spent most of her time since qualification working in clinical medicine in Oxford. She is now a Clinical Research Fellow in the Oxford Centre for Diabetes, Endocrinology and Metabolism.

Jenny Shaw

Diabetes research nurse, The Oxford Centre for Diabetes, Endocrinology and Metabolism

Jenny has been working with people with diabetes for many years, previously as a diabetes specialist nurse and currently as a diabetes research nurse. In recent years, she has been involved in studies of the development of new treatments for people with type 2 diabetes.

1

Diabetes: an overview

What is diabetes?

Diabetes is the medical condition where there is too much sugar circulating in the bloodstream. The main sugar found in the body is glucose, and it is essential for good health. The body normally regulates glucose very precisely between its normal fasting level and a concentration about double normal. Blood glucose concentrations above the normal limits for any length of time can lead to problems, so it is important that diabetes is diagnosed early and treated appropriately. The hormone that controls blood glucose is insulin, and this is normally produced in appropriate amounts in the pancreas—a large fleshy organ under the stomach that also produces many of the digestive enzymes. Insulin deficiency—either complete or partial—is the basic mechanism behind diabetes, although other factors have an influence and can sometimes be more important when considering treatment.

Different types of diabetes

Diabetes is generally divided into the categories 'type 1 diabetes' and 'type 2 diabetes'. They have much in common with each other, but differ in the cause and urgency of treatment necessary (see Table 1.1). As a broad generalization, type 1 diabetes occurs in those who are generally younger, so children and teenagers are more likely to have type 1 diabetes, and those in middle age type 2. It is also true that those with type 1 diabetes are generally of normal weight, while overweight is common in those with type 2. It is certain that overweight is a risk for type 2 diabetes, and not for type 1. Type 1 diabetes has a rapid onset, and symptoms can be quite severe. Prompt medical intervention is almost always necessary. Type 2 diabetes is quite strongly genetic (being found in families from one generation to the next, and in brothers and sisters as they get to middle age or older) and is also related to lifestyle factors such as low levels of physical activity and weight gain. Unlike type 1 diabetes, it can have a very slow and insidious onset, and the diagnosis may be missed for many months or even be found by chance on routine medical testing for other conditions. Early diagnosis is worthwhile, however, because it has been shown that complications of diabetes (discussed in detail later in this book) can be reduced and delayed by appropriate treatment.

Table 1.1 Differences between type 1 and type 2 diabetes

	Type 1 diabetes	Type 2 diabetes
Older and alternative names	Juvenile-onset diabetes Insulin-dependent diabetes mellitus (IDDM)	Maturity-onset diabetes Non-insulin-dependent diabetes mellitus (NIDDM)
Onset	Any time in life, but teenagers and children are most likely to have this type	Generally diagnosed over the age of 40, but can occur in the overweight or in some genetic conditions in younger people
Symptoms at onset	Thirst, tiredness, weight loss, passing urine very frequently, rapid breathing when the condition becomes extreme	Tiredness, passing urine more frequently, especially at night, thrush and skin infections
Body type	Generally normal weight or thin	Generally overweight
Speed of onset	Usually becomes critical and needs urgent attention within a few weeks (or even days) of the first symptoms	May not be noticed as a problem. Onset can be very slow. Sometimes just discovered by routine screening with no symptoms. Sometimes discovered because of a 'complication'
Genetics	Some genetic propensity to run in families, but not caused by a single gene	Quite a strong genetic propensity to run in families, but not caused by a single gene
Triggered by	Autoimmunity. A condition where the body mistakes the cells producing insulin for 'foreign' cells and destroys them as though they were an infection	Relative insulin deficiency where the cells making insulin do not produce sufficient amounts. Often complicated by insulin not working effectively
Treated by	Optimizing lifestyle and the use of insulin	Lifestyle change, which may initially be enough. Generally will need tablets, and probably, later, need insulin
How common	About 0.2% of the population (2 cases per 1000 people).	Up to 4% of the UK population, up to 8% in the USA, up to 20% in parts of Asia and up to 50% in some American Indians.

What causes diabetes?

Although a great deal is known about the mechanisms and the processes involved in diabetes, the exact causes of both type 1 and type 2 diabetes remain unknown. What is well understood is much about the mechanisms operating and how to alter these to advantage in order to minimize the effects of diabetes.

Normal glucose usage in the body (metabolism)

To understand diabetes, it is helpful to understand how the body functions normally to manage its energy requirements. The body can be regarded as a biological engine, and like all engines it requires fuel. However, there is a fundamental difference in the way that energy needs to be directed. In a physical engine, such as that in a car, the fuel is injected in one area. In the body, every one of the living cells needs fuel and oxygen in order to remain viable, and the circulation therefore needs to supply these requirements to many billions of cells. Normally the major fuel is glucose, though fats and protein and some other chemical entities can be utilized. Glucose comes from food digested in the gut, and some is used immediately. Most, however, is stored in the liver locked into large molecules called glycogen, and glycogen also stores glucose in the muscles ready for sudden surges of exercise. At the same time, because glucose is dangerous in high concentrations, the levels in the blood have to be controlled, and then, in contrast, in a fasting state glucose must be released from the liver in sufficient quantities to avoid the body running out of fuel. If the glucose becomes too low ('hypoglycaemia') the brain slows and then stops working. Unconsciousness follows, and, if no correction is applied, there is a risk to life itself. All this distribution and control of glucose is managed by a chemical messenger—insulin—which is secreted into the bloodstream from one cell type, the beta-cell, found in the islets of Langerhans (tight collections of differing cell types) scattered throughout the pancreas. These beta-cells monitor the prevailing glucose concentration and secrete insulin appropriately— more insulin when the glucose is high and less insulin when the glucose is low. The cells of the body pick up this insulin message—the liver and muscles will take up glucose when the insulin is high, and when the insulin is low the liver will start to release the glucose that it has stored in the glycogen molecules. The brain does not respond to insulin in the control of its fuel supply—it just needs the glucose to be present in sufficient concentration.

It follows that when the beta-cells do not work properly for any reason, the blood glucose will rise—and that is diabetes. It is also true that if the insulin does not signal properly to the cells of the body for any reason then the control mechanism will not function well. This phenomenon is called 'insulin resistance' and is also widely found in diabetes.

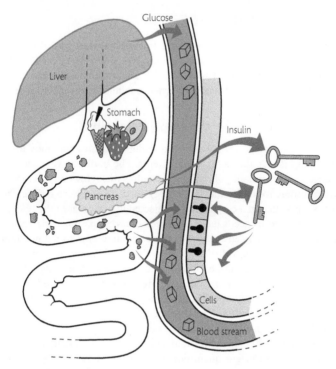

Figure 1.1 A diagram of insulin action on the body. Insulin can be regarded as a key unlocking access to cells.

Abnormal glucose usage in the body (metabolism): diabetes

As outlined above, there are two broad types of diabetes. They both involve problems with the beta-cells producing insulin, but they seem to have very different and distinctive pathologies.

In type 1 diabetes, the beta-cells are destroyed over a matter of few weeks by a mistake made by the body's immune system. The immune system has evolved to detect and destroy strange things in the body. So viruses and bacteria are wiped out, and then the body raises 'antibodies' so that the next time such a virus or bacterium appears it is eradicated extremely quickly. That is why one can usually only get measles, mumps or chicken pox once in a lifetime. Immunization depends on giving some kind of attenuated germ (dead or alive-but-weak) so that when the real thing comes along the antibodies are in place. However, the body can make mistakes—and one immune mistake is that it recognizes normal cells as being foreign, and then triggers the system for destruction. Type 1 diabetes is such an autoimmune disease. The body produces islet cell antibodies (which we can detect in the laboratory and measure) and then the beta-cells are wiped out. It can be seen from this that insulin is the only way of treating such a condition. Nothing that can stimulate beta-cells to function better will work if there are no beta-cells at all.

Type 2 diabetes, on the other hand, is characterized by a loss of function of the beta-cells, but they can still be found in the pancreas. Why don't they work? We still do not know. It may be that they have filled up with an odd protein that is similar to one found in some neurological diseases and sometimes in ageing. It may be that the nucleus stops working properly or that fat accumulates and stops the cell releasing the insulin in appropriate amounts. Much research continues to focus on this vexed question. What happens in practice is that the blood glucose gradually rises, and the rise may be so gradual that the abnormality may be present for many years before the diagnosis is made. Type 2 diabetes is also associated with insulin resistance, so that which is produced does not work as well as normal. That is then a double problem.

It can also be appreciated that there are forms of diabetes that are neither type 1 nor type 2. If the pancreas is removed surgically after an accident, destroyed by alcohol excess or affected by disease, then diabetes ensues—this is called 'secondary' diabetes. If insulin resistance increases markedly and suddenly—as it does with high-dose steroid therapy—then the signalling of insulin fails and the glucose rises to a point where diabetes is diagnosed. If the islets themselves have a missing genetic code for part of their sensing system, then glucose is not properly controlled. This diabetes type is called MODY (maturity-onset diabetes of the young). Table 1.2 outlines some of the rarer types of diabetes.

Table 1.2 Some of the rarest types of diabetes

Name of diabetes type	Caused by	Features
Surgical secondary diabetes	Pancreas removal	Diabetes occurs immediately post-operatively and insulin is always needed
Gestational diabetes	Insulin demand increasing during pregnancy	May resolve after birth of the child. Generally a marker of risk of later type 2 diabetes. Insulin needed usually during pregnancy
MODY	Genetic miscodes mainly related to the beta-cell	Several different MODY types described. Some are non-progressive forms of diabetes. Occur in 50% of all family members on average

(continued)

Table 1.2 Some of the rarest types of diabetes *(continued)*

Name of diabetes type	Caused by	Features
Drug-induced diabetes	Mainly caused by high-dose steroids	High-dose steroids are life-saving for some diseases. However, there is a risk that while on steroids diabetes will occur—likely to need insulin
Calcific diabetes	Calcium deposits in the pancreas	Rare, but can run in families
Pancreatitis-associated diabetes	Islets destroyed in an inflammatory reaction	Pancreatitis can be caused by high blood fats, alcohol excess or simply be something occurring without a trigger cause. Pancreatitis is painful and can be life-threatening
MIDD, DIDMOAD	Rare genetic syndromes	A variety of diabetes types occur—some with deafness

Ann came to England in 1945, and was diagnosed when the matron at her boarding school found her drinking the bath water

Ann   www.diabetes-stories.com

Symptoms of diabetes

Normally there is no conscious awareness of blood glucose concentrations. The levels stay within a range for normal function and do not become so high that symptoms occur. However, when the blood glucose becomes too high, a variety of symptoms will occur. The first is that the kidney removes the excess glucose from the blood and excretes it from the body in the urine. Normally there is no glucose in the urine at all, but if the blood glucose goes above about 12 mmol/l this exceeds the renal (kidney's) capacity and then glucose can be detected in the urine. The glucose brings with it a quantity of fluid, and this extra fluid leads to excessive urine production (polyuria) which may be apparent in the night (nocturia) and may in turn lead to considerable thirst (polydipsia)

At the same time, if the insulin cannot signal to the cells to take the glucose in, the paradox occurs that despite the high concentrations in the circulation the cells themselves are deprived of fuel. This has been termed 'starvation in the midst of plenty'. The starvation shows itself initially as weight loss and weakness, and can progress to extremes where someone with untreated type 1 diabetes seems to be truly clinically starving.

My symptoms were drinking all the time, which was terrible—having this terrible, terrible thirst, and no matter what you did, you could not quench this thirst. And I used to, well I used to do totally the wrong thing really because I used to drink pop—whatever I could get my hands on; water as well, because I was desperate most of the time. And then I suddenly realised that I was losing a lot of weight.

Jeanette   www.diabetes-stories.com

This is very unusual now as the diagnosis will have been made long before such serious symptoms occur.

Meanwhile, with a lack of insulin, the body switches to a reserve fuel supply—fat. Fat can normally be utilized in the absence of food without any adverse reactions, but when there is no glucose available to the cells the energy production relies on fat stores and by-products known as ketones. Ketones in small quantities can be used by the body as fuel, but in large quantities are too acidic. If the body becomes acid, this causes very rapid breathing in an attempt to remove the acid from the body. The combination of high ketone levels and acid is called ketoacidosis and is the clinical condition of type 1 diabetes completely out of control—dehydration, acidosis, rapid breathing and a sweet smell of ketones on the breath. Only emergency medical treatment can then prevent coma and ultimate death.

With type 2 diabetes such extremes of symptoms do not occur. Instead the symptoms are much more insidious. The glucose in the urine may only cause a minimal amount of polyuria, perhaps being thought of as normal. 'I have no problems—I'm only up once in the night'. Or the glucose may lead to infections in the urinary tract or in the groin. But again these may not be regarded as being serious enough to bring them to medical attention. Years of slightly raised glucose will harden up the arteries, and many people have been diagnosed with diabetes after they have had a heart attack—itself caused by the diabetes. These long-term 'tissue complications' are a problem in their own right, and are discussed in detail later in the book. They include macrovascular disease (relating to large blood vessels) which are essentially stroke, heart attack and loss of circulation to the limbs, and microvascular disease (relating to small blood vessels) which includes retinopathy (eye problems), neuropathy (loss of sensation) and nephropathy (kidney problems). All these complications of diabetes can be minimized with good control of blood glucose, blood fats and blood pressure.

A short history of diabetes

Although it has been claimed that diabetes was described in an ancient Egyptian 'Ebers papyrus' from 1500 BC, no real medical understanding of diabetes was apparent until the eighteenth century. Nevertheless the disease was seen and described: the name 'diabetes' is attributable to Demetrios of Apamaia (*c.* 150 BC) meaning a siphon or excessive fluid. It was this aspect of diabetes that was especially apparent. By about 160 AD, there was a completely recognizable description from Arateus of Cappadocia: 'diabetes is an awkward affection melting down the flesh and limbs into the urine . . . The patients never stop making water . . . Life is short and painful . . . They are affected with nausea, restlessness and a burning thirst and at no distant term they expire'. But no progress regarding the cause was made until Thomas Willis (1621–1675), working in Oxford, noted the sweet taste of urine in diabetes mellitus. By then it was clear that a disease associated with sweet urine (diagnosed by tasting it) was afflicting some overweight people. Matthew Dobson, in 1771, noted that there was excess sugar in the blood—also, alarmingly, by tasting it. In 1797, John Rollo, in an account published by the Physicians of London, recorded two cases of diabetes mellitus (luis venerea) and a trial of diet. One patient improved, the other did not. From this time onwards careful observation and recording of data became the watchword of medicine, and the scientific method grew and flourished. Then in 1890, Minkowski discovered that dogs would develop diabetes if their pancreas was surgically removed. Here was the first evidence of some effect of something produced in the pancreas that was vital to life—what was this 'something'? Meanwhile Langerhans had described 'islets' within the exocrine tissue of the pancreas, and recognized that there were a variety of cell types. Could these islets be secreting something into the circulation and, if so, what? The answer was to come from a Canadian group of Collip, McCleod, Banting and Best who were working on this problem and extracted from the pancreas something that would reverse the symptoms of diabetes in a dog that had had its pancreas removed. They had discovered the answer—a hormone that they knew came from the islets—and so they named it 'isletin' or 'insulin'. Within a year, insulin was being extracted from animal pancreas and being used successfully in man. From 1923, no-one needed to die from acute type 1 diabetes.

One should not underestimate the significance of the discovery of insulin. It was really the very first time that any scientists had achieved the full process of understanding a disease, finding a deficiency, identifying the deficiency, extracting a protein, purifying the protein, injecting the protein and establishing a clinical cure. The Nobel prize, given for this work, was richly deserved.

Then in the 1930s Hagedorn discovered that the absorption of insulin could be slowed if it was stabilized with a fish protein called protamine. Neutral Protamine Hagedorn (NPH) was the result, and has been used by many thousands since that time. Zinc could be used to slow absorption as well, and zinc insulins and mixtures of insulins soon came on the market.

Type 2 diabetes could be treated with insulin, and some years after its diagnosis many people need insulin. But until the 1950s the mainstay was weight loss and careful diet. Then, it was noted that some people on sulphonamide antibiotics had low glucose. From this observation sulphonylureas (chlorpropamide and tolbutamide) were discovered and have remained a mainstay of treatment ever since. Further clinical research led to the launch of gliclazide, and the hunt for improved efficacy resulted in the marketing of glibenclamide. Biguanides (metformin) were discovered in the 1950s and have been used widely since then.

Little changed in therapy for several decades. However, the so-called 'tissue complications' of diabetes began to be recognized in ever growing numbers of patients. Blindness was a feared tragedy, and limb amputations were not rare. Some physicians felt that keeping blood sugars as near to normal as possible would minimize these complications, but there was no strong evidence for this.

Then, in the 1970s, things began to change. It was discovered that eye disease (retinopathy) could be treated by laser therapy. At last there was a specific treatment and, in most cases, a cure for advancing eye disease.

Therapeutics was advancing too. Novo, a Danish company that had been producing insulin from the early days, produced the first really pure preparation of insulin—'monocomponent insulin'—which helped to prevent some of the local complications of insulin injection.

By the late 1970s diabetes was still being treated with a very narrow range of products—metformin and sulphonylureas for early type 2 diabetes and insulin for type 1 and late type 2. But no-one had answered the fundamental question about whether trying to keep the blood glucose near normal led to improved outcome compared with a more relaxed policy. During the 1990s this question was answered with the publication of two large clinical trials, one in type 1 diabetes (the Diabetes Control and Complications Trial or DCCT) and one in type 2 diabetes (the United Kingdom Prospective Diabetes Study or UKPDS), and both showed that intensive treatment to lower blood glucose levels improved outcomes. The UKPDS also showed that lowering blood pressure had a positive impact on health.

Meanwhile, for type 2 diabetes, pharmaceutical companies, using the newly emergent understanding of protein chemistry, began to hunt for chemical 'targets' in the body. The body's lack of response to insulin came under scrutiny and by the 1990s thiazolidinediones were being designed and tested. New sulphonylureas had already been pioneered (glimepiride), and then two short-acting compounds were marketed (repaglinide and nateglinide). Agents for slowing food absorption, and for slowing the progression of complications were the subject of a growing number of clinical trials.

Further breakthroughs in the understanding of the detailed physiology of the beta-cell were fundamental to the next generation of agents. The beta-cell in the islets of Langerhans had a known structure when fixed under the microscope, but how did it work? All that was known until late into the twentieth century was 'glucose in→insulin out'. A so-called 'black box'. But soon new scientific techniques and astonishing technology led to the recognition of a large number of pathways inside the cell. The cell turned out to be a small city of inter-relating mechanisms, even with its own internal railway lines and trucking working by energy supplied from the glucose absorbed. Now there was more information for many more targets—new surface 'receptors' (signal stations) were discovered, some being activated by chemical messengers which we recognized and some receptors having no known activator at all. These 'orphan' receptors have come under scrutiny along with all the molecular targets that could be manipulated in the islets, liver and brain, muscle and fat cells of the body. The complex array of agents now available is a testimony to dedicated research.

Treatment of diabetes

The treatment of diabetes will be discussed in some detail in Chapter 3, but the principles are straightforward. Maintaining blood glucose levels as near to the normal range as possible reduces the risk of long-term complications. In type 1 diabetes there is a need to manipulate insulin in order to get the glucose in a safe working range, and this range varies from individual to individual. Blood fats will generally need to be lowered, and 'statins' are widely prescribed to achieve this. The large studies have shown that there are fewer complications if the blood pressure is reduced—even slightly below normal. Typically, in type 2 diabetes, patients will find themselves on several agents for blood pressure: a statin, glucose-lowering therapy and perhaps aspirin. Is all this necessary? The answer is that large clinical trials have shown that this approach to therapy is the way of maintaining health and freedom from complications for many years. This is called the 'evidence base', and the evidence continues to accumulate year on year.

How common is diabetes?

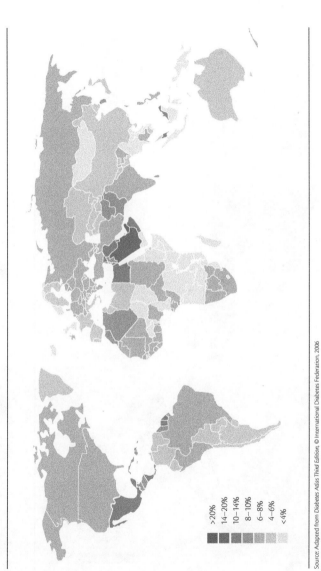

>20%
14–20%
10–14%
8–10%
6–8%
4–6%
<4%

Source: Adapted from *Diabetes Atlas Third Edition*, © International Diabetes Federation, 2006

Figure 1.2 Prevalence estimates of diabetes, 2007.

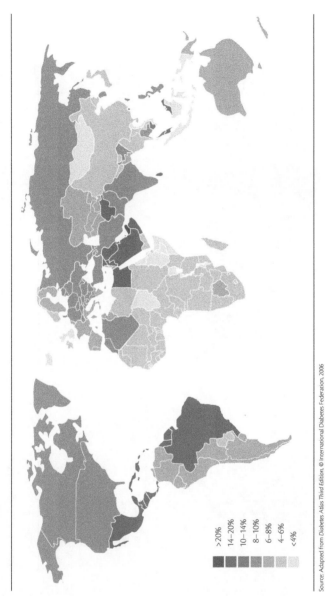

Source: Adapted from *Diabetes Atlas Third Edition*, © International Diabetes Federation, 2006

Figure 1.3 Prevalence estimates of diabetes, 2025.

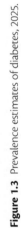

>20%
14–20%
10–14%
8–10%
6–8%
4–6%
<4%

Diabetes worldwide

Type 2 diabetes is reaching epidemic proportions in all parts of the world. The figures produced from the World Health Organization demonstrate that in the UK we have moved from a prevalence of about 2% to about 4% in just a decade or two. In the USA, the rates are double this, and in some parts of the developing world rates of up to 20% are being reported in urban communities.

Figure 1.4 shows the trend in the USA, reflected in many other parts of the world where the rates of diabetes are doubling or trebling over one or two decades.

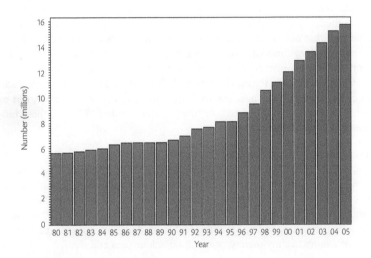

Figure 1.4 Diabetes trends in the USA.

The scale and the time course of the epidemic demonstrate that this is an environmental issue (no genetic basis can cause a tripling of a disease over 20 years), but there is a strong genetic *tendency*—in other words diabetes runs in families. But as with all epidemics, interventions are possible. The environment can be changed—but the changes need to be widespread, and relate to improving lifestyles. There is a need to be serious about food consumption and food labelling, about urban design for exercise on a daily basis, about building design where stairs become the norm and lifts are hidden away, about playgrounds for children, about the couch-potato mentality of computer games and hours of inactive television viewing. There is a need to reach out to communities where diabetes is devastating their present and future health and work towards an equitable sharing of the world's resources. Malnutrition in the world is widespread. But malnutrition has two ends of its spectrum. Many in the world have too little to eat. On the other hand there is a developed society malnutrition of eating too much of the wrong kinds of food. This is a problem of societies: governments and healthcare providers need to act decisively on a wide range of issues to prevent millions of people being disadvantaged by a prevalent but inappropriate lifestyle.

Diabetes as an ongoing disease

Diabetes is not curable at the moment. But it is neither a disaster nor a death sentence. Most people with diabetes will need to monitor what is happening to their blood glucose and will need to concentrate carefully on taking appropriate medication—including insulin—at the right time. Everyone should be aware of what needs surveillance (eyes, feet, heart, glucose, blood fats, blood pressure, kidney function, and nerve function), and it is reasonable to take a proper and lively interest in what the numbers on the desk of the healthcare professionals actually mean. Those with diabetes should ask for the results and an explanation of their meaning each time there is a review. Is more, less or different medication, treatment or investigation needed? What do these biochemical measurements imply?

It is reasonable to encourage all those with diabetes to get involved in trying to stop the epidemic and in helping everyone towards a better life. Research is a high priority if prevention and treatment are to be improved. Diabetes could be cured if we understood more of the science of the mechanisms of failure of insulin secretion in the body. There are many ways to get involved: talking to those who organize and pay for services, community activities for the promotion of a more healthy society, research questionnaires and trials.

I also feel fairly positive about the future, because I really do believe we've seen enough changes over 20 years to expect that the life of diabetics is going to improve beyond belief, that my daughter's future is much brighter than even mine, and I don't feel despondent about mine.

Gillian   www.diabetes-stories.com

2

Lifestyle

Introduction

> . . . I have always thought that diabetes is no big deal. But then I start thinking about the amount of time I spend every single day thinking about it: thinking about, you know, what my blood sugars are, how they're going to be affected by doing certain things—if I go swimming, well, you know, where will I have lunch? Will my sugars go too low? Have I got glucose on me? How to work out the certain amount of carbohydrate if we go out for a meal. You know, you do spend an awful lot of your time thinking about it, and it's so much part of you, though, that you're not even aware.
>
> Clare   type 1 diabetes

Managing diabetes can be challenging and time-consuming as it requires attention to everyday activities including food and physical activity, and investigating and reflecting upon their effects on blood glucose levels. Diabetes is a condition that is greatly affected by lifestyle choices in everyday life; eating a large meal will have more effect on blood glucose levels than eating a small snack, taking part in physical activity can lower glucose levels, losing weight will have a positive effect on both overall health and blood glucose levels. Self-management of these lifestyle factors influences outcomes in both the long and the short term. There is much confusion about the ideal diet for diabetes, about how much physical activity people should engage in and how other aspects of their life affect blood glucose levels. These issues are all addressed in this lifestyle chapter.

You know, you're really very fit as a diabetic. You actually have a very, very good diet, a healthy diet and you're encouraged to take exercise, which I did.

Ann   type 1 diabetes

There is nothing to be afraid of, as long as you eat sensibly, exercise sensibly, you can live your lifespan just like any normal person.

George   type 1 diabetes

Diet

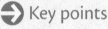 **Key points**

* Diet can help control blood glucose levels and prevent heart disease and stroke.

* Starchy and sugary carbohydrate foods have most effect on blood glucose after eating.

* Reducing total fat and salt intake can help reduce the risk of heart disease and stroke.

* Fruit and vegetables are an important part of a healthy diet and increasing intake can help reduce the risk of heart disease and some cancers.

Food is one of the most important factors affecting blood glucose, and influences health in two ways: by the type of food eaten (the quality of the diet) and the amount of food eaten (the quantity of the diet). Managing food intake can help:

* regulate blood glucose levels,

* reduce the risk of heart disease and stroke,

* weight management.

In the UK, Diabetes UK (the charity for people with diabetes) has published nutritional recommendations for people with diabetes. These recommendations are theoretical and given in terms of nutrients, rather than foods, and for this reason are not reproduced here. Guidelines for diabetes are designed to regulate blood glucose levels and provide an overall healthy diet. A practical summary of the dietary guidelines is given below.

Practical dietary guidelines for people with diabetes

◆ Eat regularly. For some people this may mean three times a day, others may find they need snacks between meals. Eating large meals at irregular intervals can cause blood glucose levels to rise significantly after meals, and many people eat more than they need if they have gone for long periods without food.

◆ Include some starchy carbohydrate foods at each meal. Starchy foods are digested to glucose and raise blood glucose levels and provide energy. Sugary carbohydrate foods can be included in the diet of people with diabetes, but they contain less minerals and vitamins than starchy foods, and large quantities will cause weight gain and high blood glucose levels.

◆ Adopt a low fat diet. High intakes of fat, especially saturated (animal) fat, are associated with weight gain and heart disease.

◆ Reduce salt and salty foods. High salt intakes can lead to high blood pressure, a risk factor for heart disease.

◆ Eat at least five portions of fruit and vegetables every day. These foods contain vitamins, minerals and fibre, and are an important part of a healthy diet. There is evidence that they can help prevent heart disease and some cancers.

Blood glucose management

The main type of nutrient in food that affects blood glucose levels is called carbohydrate, often referred to as 'carbs'. Most foods contain a mixture of fat, protein and carbohydrate, but foods containing mainly protein and fat have a minimal effect on blood glucose levels compared with carbohydrate-containing foods. Carbohydrates are found mainly in starchy and sugary foods. All carbohydrates are digested into glucose and appear in the bloodstream between 10 minutes and 2 hours or more after eating.

Most foods are a mixture of protein, fat and carbohydrate.

Table 2.1 Examples of foods in each food group

Food group	Role in the body	Example foods
Protein	Tissue growth and repair	Meat, poultry, fish, eggs, cheese, nuts, soya products, pulses (lentils, dried beans and peas)
Fat	Energy and structure	Butter, margarine, all vegetable oils (olive, corn, sunflower), cream, lard, suet
Carbohydrate	Energy	Starchy foods, sugary foods, fruit, milk

Protein foods alone will have little effect on blood glucose levels, but some protein foods do have carbohydrate added during processing. This may be cereal or flour (sauces, sausages), breadcrumbs (fish fingers, chicken nuggets) or pastry (meat pie, pasties, quiche, sausage rolls).

Fat has little effect on glucose levels after eating, but large amounts can slow the digestion of a meal and cause a more gradual rise in blood glucose levels. Examples of high fat food meals which may have this effect include fish and chips, hamburger and fries, and take-away meals such as Chinese or Indian foods made with large quantities of oil or fat.

All carbohydrate foods are digested to glucose and will have the greatest effect on blood levels after eating. They include all starchy and sugary foods (see Figure 2.1).

Which foods contain carbohydrate?

Table 2.2 Foods that raise blood glucose levels after eating (carbohydrate foods)

Starchy foods	◆ Rice, pasta, noodles, bread (all types—wholemeal, white, French, pitta, naan bread), breakfast cereals, grains (couscous, bulgur wheat), flour (in pastry, sauces, pizza bases), plain biscuits and crackers and starchy vegetables (potato, yam, sweet potato, lentils, dried peas and beans)
Sugary foods	◆ Any food made with ordinary sugar (sucrose) contains carbohydrate. These foods include cakes, biscuits, chocolate, sweets, jam, honey, marmalade, puddings, desserts, squashes and fizzy drinks
	◆ Fruit contains natural sugar (fructose). Fruit (e.g. apples, oranges, bananas, melon, mango) and fruit juice (both 'natural' or 'unsweetened' and sweetened) contain carbohydrate
	◆ Milk and yoghurt contain natural sugar (lactose). All milk, whether full-cream, semi-skimmed, skimmed, pasteurized, homogenized or long-life, and products made from milk (e.g. custard and ice-cream) contain carbohydrate

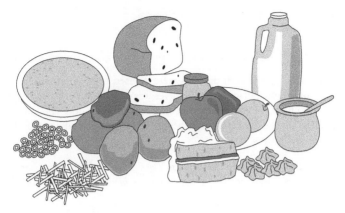

Figure 2.1 Carbohydrate-containing food.

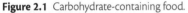

Different foods contain different amounts of carbohydrate and will have different effects on blood glucose levels. Carbohydrate foods are an important source of energy in the diet, and glucose is a vital fuel for many tissues in the body and especially the brain. The challenge for many people with diabetes is eating an amount of carbohydrate that meets their energy demands without causing high blood glucose levels.

? FAQ

How do I know if I'm eating the right amount of carbohydrate?

The amount of food and carbohydrate eaten is very individual. If your weight is stable and your blood glucose levels are within target, you're probably eating the right amount. Some people find that measuring their blood glucose levels after eating can be helpful in working out the effect of different foods.

❌ Myth

People with diabetes should avoid sugar and sugary foods.

Traditionally, people with diabetes were advised to avoid all foods containing sugar, and a diagnosis of diabetes was usually accompanied by the instruction never to eat sweets, chocolate, cakes, and puddings. This had a big effect on the quality of most people's life and especially on children with type 1 diabetes.

I think it was, for me, that sugar wasn't going to be allowed any more; no more sweets, no more cakes, no more icing on birthday cake, that kind of thing.

Emma   type 1 diabetes

. . . I could have no sugar at all, no sweets, nothing. And that's terrible, because all your friends are having sweets . . .

Patsy   type 1 diabetes

More recent research done on the effects of different kinds of foods on blood glucose levels has shown that sugar and starch have similar effects if they contain the same amount of carbohydrate. For example, a medium apple, a medium slice of bread and a small Kit-Kat all contain similar amounts of carbohydrate and will have a similar effect on blood glucose levels. The advice given to people with diabetes no longer recommends avoiding all sugar, but states that including small amounts of sugar in the diet will not compromise blood glucose control. Large amounts of sugary foods are not recommended for anyone, whether they have diabetes or not, and this advice is especially important for people who are trying to lose weight.

❓ FAQ

I've heard of carbohydrate counting—what is it?

Carbohydrate counting is a system usually used by people with type 1 diabetes. They calculate the total amount of carbohydrate in a meal or snack, regardless of whether it is starch or sugar, and then inject insulin to match the carbohydrate they have eaten. This system has been shown to increase flexibility in the diet and improve blood glucose control. It is used in many diabetes centres in the UK and is often delivered as part of a structured education programme. One well-known example is DAFNE (Dose Adjustment for Normal Eating), although there are now many different programmes available around the country. People with type 1 diabetes are advised to ask their health professionals for details of local course.

Carbohydrates and the glycaemic index (GI)

People with diabetes are often encouraged to adopt a low GI diet. The glycaemic index (GI) is a ranking of carbohydrate foods based on their overall effect upon blood glucose levels compared with a reference food—usually glucose or white bread. The GI of a food can only be measured in the laboratory by feeding a sample of the food to volunteers and measuring the changes in blood glucose levels. There are many factors affecting the GI of a food, including the kind of starch present, the physical make-up of the food, the amount and type of fibre present and the amount of fat and protein eaten with the food. It is impossible to guess the GI of a food—for example, chocolate milk shake has a low GI and baked potatoes are high GI.

High GI foods cause large fluctuations in blood glucose levels and

Low GI foods cause smaller fluctuations in blood glucose levels and are recommended for people with diabetes.

Foods are usually categorized as high, medium and low GI.

What do the numbers mean?

The GI value of a food is related to a number which compares the food with glucose. Glucose is given a value of 100, so the higher the value of a food, the higher the GI.

GI ranking	GI value
Low	Less than 55
Medium	56–69
High	70 or more

Table 2.3 Examples of low, medium, and high GI foods

Food	Low GI (less than 55)	Medium GI (56–69)	High GI (70 or more)
Bread	Multigrain, granary, rye	Wholemeal pitta bread	Wholemeal, brown, white, French stick, naan bread
Breakfast cereals	All-Bran, Special K, muesli, porridge	Bran cereals (Bran Flakes, Sultana Bran, Raisin Bran)	All other cereals (corn flakes, rice cereals, Shredded Wheat, Weetabix, sugared cereals)
Potatoes	Sweet potatoes, yam	New potatoes	Old potatoes— boiled, baked, mashed, roast, chips
Pasta and rice	All types of pasta, egg noodles	Basmati rice, rice noodles	Brown and white rice, rice pasta
Vegetables	Lentils and dried beans, baked beans, peas, sweetcorn		
Fruit	Apples, pears, peaches, cherries, apricots, plums, oranges, strawberries	Tropical fruit (melons, pineapple, bananas, mango)	
Dairy products	All milk (full-fat, semi-skimmed, skimmed)	Ice cream	
Cakes and biscuits	Plain sponge cake, fruit and malt bread	Digestives, Rich Tea biscuits, crackers	Doughnuts, scones
Savoury snacks	Maize and corn chips, cashew and peanuts	Crisps	Extruded potato snacks (hoops, rings, tubes) and pretzels

❓ FAQ

I see that peanuts and some cakes are low GI—does that mean I can eat lots of these foods?

The GI gives you information about how these foods will affect blood glucose levels compared with other foods, but there are other things to consider.

The amount of carbohydrate in food has more overall effect on blood glucose than the type of carbohydrate eaten, so lots of cake (even if it is low GI) will raise blood glucose levels. Peanuts will have little or no effect on blood glucose levels, but are very high in fat and energy, so if weight loss is an issue, peanuts may hinder this. Overall, if you wish to adopt a low GI diet, try to substitute the low or medium GI foods for the higher GI choices.

Is it just about the GI value—aren't there other things in the diet that affect blood glucose levels?

The GI is a relatively new concept and, as more research is done, other factors have been discovered. Mashed potato is high GI, but adding cheese to it lowers the GI. Similarly, putting tuna, baked beans or cheese onto a baked potato turns a high GI meal into a low GI meal. And adding vinegar to foods lowers the GI, so putting vinegar on your chips will lower the GI!

Glycaemic load

The GI gives an indication of the effect of different foods containing the same amount of carbohydrate, but the amount of carbohydrate eaten is equally important. A measure of GI and amount of food eaten is called the glycaemic load (GL). The GL is an attempt to give an indication of the overall effect of the food. Spaghetti, for example, is low GI but, if eaten in large amounts, can have a large effect on blood glucose. Watermelon may be high GI, but contains little carbohydrate so will have less effect on blood glucose levels. Many people find the concept of GL very confusing and, as it requires a mathematical formula to calculate, it can be impractical to use in everyday life.

Top tips for a healthy, low GI diet

- Use breakfast cereals based on oats, barley, and bran.
- Use breads made with whole grains, stone-ground, or rye flour.
- Reduce the amount of potatoes you eat.
- Enjoy all other types of fruit and vegetables.
- Use pasta and noodles.
- Use Basmati rice.
- Eat plenty of salad vegetables with a vinaigrette dressing.

> ### ➲ Key points: blood glucose management and carbohydrate
>
> ◆ Carbohydrate foods (starchy and sugary foods) have the most effect on blood glucose levels after eating.
>
> ◆ The total amount of carbohydrate present in the food predicts blood glucose levels, not whether the food contains sugar or starch.
>
> ◆ People with diabetes can include sugar in their diet, but general healthy eating advice applies and large amounts are not recommended.
>
> ◆ People with type 1 diabetes can learn a system of carbohydrate counting to increase the flexibility in their diet.

Reducing the risk of heart disease and stroke

Blood glucose control is one aspect of the management of diabetes, but diabetes is also a risk factor for heart disease and stroke, and diet can play a part in reducing this risk. The main components of the diet that affect heart health are fat and salt.

Fat

High fat intakes, particularly of animal (saturated) fat, are linked with a higher level of cholesterol in the blood and in turn with an increased risk of heart disease.

> ### ❓ FAQ
>
> #### What is cholesterol?
>
> Cholesterol is a fat-like substance that is needed in small amounts in the body. Excess cholesterol can build up in the blood vessels and affect the flow of blood. If this happens in the small blood vessels supplying the heart, then the heart cannot receive enough oxygen from the blood and this can cause pain (angina) and eventually a heart attack.

It is recommended that people with diabetes adopt a low fat diet in order to reduce this risk.

❓ FAQ

What can I do to reduce my fat intake?

You can reduce your fat intake by making changes to the way that food is cooked and by choosing lower fat versions of different foods:

- Try grilling, steaming, boiling, casseroling, and dry-roasting food rather than frying or roasting in added fat.

- Spread butter or margarine more thinly; you may find that you can stop using it altogether.

- Include less fat in foods by reducing the amount of cream, salad dressings, grated cheese, sauces, butter, margarine, or oil added to recipes.

- Pastries, pies, processed, and convenience foods can be high in fat—check the label.

- Many take-away foods are deep-fried and high in fat; try to choose dishes that have been grilled, steamed, stewed, or stir-fried.

- Substitute lower fat versions of high fat foods—see top tips below.

Table 2.4 Top tips for reducing fat intake

Food group	Instead of ...	Choose ...
Dairy foods	Full fat milk	Semi-skimmed or skimmed milk
	Full fat hard cheese such as Cheddar, Stilton, Parmesan, cream cheese	Lower fat cheeses such as Edam, Camembert, Brie, reduced fat Cheddar, cottage cheese
	Full fat yoghurt, cream	Low fat or diet yoghurt
Oils and fats	Butter or full fat margarine	Low fat butter or spreads
	Blended vegetable oils, lard, suet	Small amounts of olive, rapeseed, canola, corn, or sunflower oil

(continued)

Food group	Instead of . . .	Choose . . .
Meat, poultry, fish, and vegetarian equivalents	Fatty cuts of beef, pork, lamb	Lean cuts of beef, lamb, and pork, all game (venison, rabbit, hare)
	Poultry with skin	Chicken, turkey, duck and goose without skin, all game birds (pheasant, partridge, mallard)
	Paté, sausage rolls, meat pies and pasties, luncheon, and processed meats	Ham, lean cooked meat, low fat sausages, chicken roll
	Streaky bacon	Lean back bacon
	Fried fish in batter or breadcrumbs	All fish, steamed, grilled, or canned
	Vegetable pies and pasties, quiches, and fried vegetarian products. Nut rissoles, roasts, and bakes	Quorn products, tofu and soya bean products, lentil and bean burgers and loaves
Cakes and biscuits	Cream-filled cakes and buns, doughnuts, cakes with butter cream, shortbread, sweet and chocolate-coated biscuits	Plain low fat sponge cake, scones, fruit bread and loaves, plain biscuits (Garibaldi, Rich Tea, fig rolls)
Snacks	Crisps, potato snacks, nuts	Olives, bread sticks, crudites

Most fruit and vegetables are naturally low in fat. Starchy foods (breakfast cereals, pasta, rice, bread, and potatoes) are also low in fat, but this depends on cooking methods. Boiled and baked potatoes, for example, contain very little fat, but chips and mashed potato made with butter and cream may be very high in fat. Bread contains little fat, but toast dripping with butter has a high fat content.

❓ FAQ

I've heard that there are different kinds of fat—good and bad. Is this true?

Fat can be divided into three different types:

- Saturated (animal) fat. Found in fatty meat, butter, hard cheese, lard, suet, ghee. These fats raise cholesterol levels.

- Polyunsaturated fats. Found in corn, sunflower, and soya oil. These fats lower 'bad' cholesterol levels, but they also lower 'good' cholesterol.

- Monounsaturated fats. Found in olive oil, walnut oil, rapeseed oil, and avocados. They lower cholesterol, especially 'bad' cholesterol.

Omega-3 fat is a particular kind of polyunsaturated fat. Found in fish oil and oily fish such as salmon, herring, mackerel, sardines, pilchards, and trout. Helps prevent blood clotting and reduces triglycerides levels.

Monounsaturated and omega-3 fats are usually referred to as the 'good' fats and saturated fat as the 'bad' fat.

Salt

In addition to high fat intakes, high salt intakes are also a risk factor for heart disease. People who have a lot of salt in their diet are more likely to have high blood pressure, which increases the risk of heart disease. It is the sodium in salt that causes high blood pressure.

❗ Fact

In the UK, average intakes of salt are approximately 10 g per person per day.

Recommended intakes are 6 g per person per day—although the body only needs 1 g for health.

Lower salt intakes by reducing or avoiding the following:

- Salt added at the table or used in cooking,

- Stock cubes, soy sauce, yeast or meat-based savoury spreads,

- Cheese and cheese spreads,

- Savoury snacks (crisps, salted nuts, olives in brine),

- Canned soups, vegetables, fish, and meat,

- Many convenience ready-to-eat meals,

◆ Smoked or cured meat and fish (smoked salmon and mackerel, bacon, ham, salami),

◆ Bread, some breakfast cereals and biscuits can be high in salt—check the label.

---

❶ Fact

About three-quarters of the salt that we eat comes from processed or manufactured foods. The most effective way to reduce salt intake is to try to eat as many unprocessed, home-prepared foods as possible.

❓ FAQ

When I check food labels it mentions sodium and not salt. What does this mean?

Food manufacturers often list the sodium rather than the salt content of a food. To convert the sodium into salt you need to multiply the figure by 2.5

Example: A large 12 inch cheese and tomato pizza provides 3.6 g of sodium. 3.6 multiplied by 2.5 equals 9. So, this pizza contains 9 g of salt—one and a half times the recommended maximum of 6 g.

➡ Key points: reducing the risk of heart disease and stroke

◆ High fat intakes, especially saturated fat, are associated with high blood cholesterol levels.

◆ High salt intakes are associated with high blood pressure.

◆ Both high cholesterol levels and high blood pressure are risk factors for heart disease and stroke.

◆ Reducing fat and salt in the diet can reduce the risk of heart disease and stroke.

Fruit and vegetables

Fruit and vegetables are part of a healthy diet. There is growing evidence that people who eat a lot of fruit and vegetables develop less heart disease and cancer. In addition, fruit and vegetables provide vitamins, minerals, and substances known as phytochemicals and antioxidants that can help prevent heart disease.

> **❓ FAQ**
>
> **I know I should eat more fruit and veg, but I really don't like them. Can't I take vitamin tablets or supplements instead?**
>
> Interestingly, it seems that taking vitamins and minerals in fruit and vegetable form has a positive effect on health, and this effect is lost if the same vitamins are taken as tablets. An extensive review of vitamin and mineral supplements has shown bad news for smokers—they actually increase the risk of lung cancer by taking certain vitamins. At present, the advice remains—eat your five a day!

Five a day

It is recommended that people eat a variety of fruit and vegetables; aiming for five portions a day. Fresh, frozen, canned, juices, and dried fruit and vegetables all count towards a portion. A portion is equivalent to 80 g (about 3 oz). Potatoes and potato products are classed as starchy foods and do not contribute to fruit and vegetable intake.

The table below gives some indication of the amount of fruit and vegetables in one portion.

Vegetable type	Amount	Fruit type	Amount
Broccoli, cauliflower	2 florets	Apple, pear, banana, orange, peach	1 medium
Peas, sweetcorn, dried beans and peas, baked beans	3 heaped tablespoons	Satsumas, clementines, tangerines	2
Cabbage, spinach, kale	3 heaped tablespoons	Plums, apricots	2
Carrots, parsnips, swede	3 heaped tablespoons	Grapes	1 handful

(continued)

Vegetable type	Amount	Fruit type	Amount
Mixed salad	1 cereal bowl	Strawberries, raspberries, and other berries	1 small dessert bowl
Tomatoes	2 medium sized (raw), 3 tablespoons (canned)	Canned fruit	2 heaped tablespoons
Courgette, aubergine	Half a large vegetable	Dried fruit	1 tablespoon
Tomato, carrot and vegetables juices	1 medium glass	Orange, pineapple and fruit juices	1 medium glass

! Fact

Fruit contains natural sugar and will raise blood glucose levels. People with diabetes who eat large amounts of fruit in a short space of time will find that their blood glucose levels may rise significantly. Vegetables contain much less carbohydrate than fruit and can be eaten in larger amounts.

Physical activity

→ Key points

- Physical activity is beneficial for diabetes and general health.

- It is recommended that everyone takes part in moderate activity on most days of the week.

- Checking with a health professional before starting a rigorous exercise programme is advisable.

- People with type 1 diabetes should refer to their healthcare team for specific advice about insulin adjustment before exercise.

. . . in a lot of ways, it's (diabetes) made me healthier, because it's made me stick to a reasonable diet and it's taught me about going for exercise every day.

Shirley   type 1 diabetes

> . . . that one of the most important things I think that diabetics should do is . . . exercise. It keeps you a lot happier and keeps you in a lot better condition.
>
> Victor   type 1 diabetes

Daily physical activity is promoted for everyone, whether they have diabetes or not, as part of a healthy lifestyle.

❓ FAQ

I keep being told to increase my activity—why is this?

Regular activity can benefit you by:

- Making the insulin you produce or inject work more efficiently to help lower blood glucose levels.

- Lowering your blood pressure and blood cholesterol level and reducing your risk of heart disease.

- Helping weight management—being physically active helps you avoid weight gain and helps weight loss when combined with eating less.

- Making you feel better. Activity raises chemicals in your brain called endorphins and serotonin—these are often referred to as the 'feel good' hormones.

Many people think that increasing their physical activity means they must go to the gym or take up running or some sport. Although this may be enjoyable and feasible for some, it may not suit everyone. Some people are happy to dedicate some specific time to an activity each day, and others find that just increasing their activity in their everyday life can be effective. Everyday activities that can increase overall fitness include housework, gardening, cycling, DIY, and walking the dog.

❓ FAQ

How much physical activity do I need to do?

It is recommended that you try to be moderately physically active for 30 minutes on at least 5 days, and preferably every day, of the week. Two periods of 15 minutes or three periods of 10 minutes can make up the total 30 minutes.

What does moderate activity mean?

A moderately physical activity is one that makes you breathe harder than usual (but not so hard that you can't hold a conversation), where you are aware of your heart beating harder than usual or where you begin to sweat. For many people, brisk walking is a moderate activity.

So, if I decide to take up walking—how far do I need to go?

You can decide to walk for a specific period of time each day, or you can think about the distance you wish to walk. Some people find that using a pedometer is helpful. A pedometer is a simple device attached to your waistband or belt that measures how many steps you take.

How many steps should I take?

The recommendation is 10,000 steps a day. Measuring your usual daily activity will show you how much activity you take each day, and you can then set realistic targets to increase your activity. Any increase above your normal activity will improve your health.

Physical activity and type 1 diabetes

People with type 1 diabetes can find managing physical activity challenging. Balancing insulin therapy and food can help to reduce the risk of hypoglycaemia (hypos), maintain blood glucose levels and maximize performance.

Planning ahead for exercise can help, and testing blood glucose levels before, during and after exercise can provide information about individual response to exercise. Insulin doses and food intake may need some adjustment before exercise. It is recommended that people with type 1 diabetes who wish to increase their physical activity should discuss this with their healthcare team.

What affects blood glucose levels during exercise?

High blood glucose levels may be caused by the following:

- If there is a shortage of insulin, glucose cannot enter the muscle cells and the blood glucose level will rise.

- The body recognizes an increased need for glucose to provide energy and will release glucose from the liver stores. This will raise blood glucose levels.

Low blood glucose levels may be caused by the following:

- Glucose is used by the muscles to provide energy during exercise and this causes blood glucose levels to fall.

- Insulin may be absorbed more quickly than usual from the injection site if the blood supply to that area is increased by exercise.

Why can hypos be more difficult to detect during exercise?

Many of the recognized symptoms of a hypo are often experienced during normal exercise, for instance feeling hot or sweaty and noticing an increased heart rate. Checking blood glucose levels provides information to make the necessary adjustments in insulin or food intake. A previous hypo during the last 24 hours may increase the risk of further hypos, and this risk is further increased by exercise.

❓ FAQ

What exercise should I choose?

Whilst any exercise is beneficial, you should choose an activity that best meets your goals and is safe for you to do. There are two types of exercise: aerobic and anaerobic.

What is aerobic exercise?

During aerobic exercise, plenty of oxygen is available to the muscles, allowing them to use glucose and fats completely to provide energy. Examples of aerobic activity are running, jogging, using a treadmill or rowing machine, and cycling. Prolonged aerobic activity at low intensity is best for weight control.

What is anaerobic exercise?

Anaerobic exercise starts when there is not enough oxygen supplied to the muscles. Typically, anaerobic exercise occurs when you do short bursts of intense activity such as sprinting or weight training. You may find that you do not need to take extra glucose or reduce your insulin dose for this type of exercise.

Is it safe for me to exercise?

Exercise is vital to staying fit and healthy. Before starting a new exercise regimen, you may wish to discuss insulin adjustment with your diabetes team. This will be particularly important if you have complications of diabetes that affect your feet, heart, eyes, or blood pressure.

Top tips for exercising safely with type 1 diabetes

- Test blood glucose levels before, during and after exercise.

- Before exercise: aim for blood glucose levels between 6 and 13 mmol/l. If blood glucose is less than 6 mmol/l, take some fast-acting carbohydrate (jelly beans, banana, glucose tablets, soft drink, sports drink) to raise blood glucose levels. If glucose is above 13 mmol/l, either delay exercise or take some fast-acting insulin. Discuss this with your healthcare team.

- During exercise, keep some fast-acting carbohydrate handy to treat any hypoglycaemia. If you take part in prolonged or endurance exercise, you will need to take some extra carbohydrate to provide the necessary energy. It is recommended that you discuss this with a specialist healthcare professional.

- After exercise, replace liver glucose stores by eating a carbohydrate-rich meal within an hour of activity.

Weight management

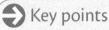 Key points

- Weight loss for those individuals who are overweight or obese has a beneficial effect on overall health and blood glucose control.

- There is not one ideal way to achieve weight loss, the key lies with finding the most effective approach for each individual.

- Losses of between 5 and 10% of starting weight can have beneficial effects.

- Weight maintenance requires long-term, realistic lifestyle changes.

Being overweight or obese has an effect on quality of life and health in people with and without diabetes. Weight reduction is routinely advised for all people whose weight falls outside the healthy range.

? FAQ

How do I know if my weight is outside the healthy range?

The body mass index (BMI) is commonly used to measure normal weight, overweight and obesity. To work out your BMI it's best to use a calculator.

BMI = your weight in kilograms divided by your height in metres squared. This can be written as a formula:

Weight (kg)/(height (m) × height (m))

So, I weigh 12 stones and I am 5ft 6 inches tall—what's my BMI?

First you need to convert stones to kilograms and feet and inches to metric measurements. 12 stones are 76.3 kg and 5ft 6 inches is 1.68 m. The formula would look like this:

76.3/1.68 × 1.68 = 27.0

That means my BMI is 27, but am I overweight?

The table below tells you what your BMI means. Different levels of BMI pose different risks in ethnic groups.

Classification	BMI	
	White Caucasian	Asian
Underweight	Less than 18.4	Less than 18.4
Normal range	18.5–24.9	18.5–22.9
Overweight	25–29.9	23–24.9
Obese	30–39.9	25–34.9
Morbidly obese	Over 40	Over 35

This means that I am overweight—am I at any risk?

Health risks increase with increasing BMI. You can reduce risk by losing weight and reducing your BMI. Assessing risk is not just about BMI; there is a lot of evidence that your waist measurement is important. A high waist measurement (circumference) suggests that there is a lot of fat in the abdomen and this kind of fat is more dangerous to health than the kind of fat that is found under the skin around the hips and thighs.

What should my waist circumference be?

For women, waist circumference should be below 80 cm (31.5 inches). White and black men should have a waist circumference below 94 cm (37 inches), and the cut-off point for Asian men is 90 cm (35 inches).

Weight reduction for overweight and obese people with diabetes has an enormous impact on overall health and diabetes. The benefits of weight loss include:

- Feeling and looking better.

- Improved blood glucose levels.

- Overall reduction in risk of cardiovascular disease and cancer.

- Improved ability to take part in physical activity.

Although most people who are overweight are aware that their health would benefit from weight loss, achieving this can be very challenging. Many people have repeated attempts at weight loss and feel disheartened when they fail to achieve their long-term goal of maintaining a healthy weight.

> . . . and it took me, as I say, quite a few months to actually start losing weight, but I managed to do it. And I reduced the amount of food I was eating and I managed to lose between two and two and two and a half stone
>
> Mary   type 1 diabetes

Getting started

Losing weight can only be achieved by taking in less energy than is expended. This can be accomplished through diet alone, by increasing physical activity, or a combination of the two. Many people are aware of the changes they may need to make in order to reduce their weight, but find executing the changes very demanding. Balancing medication, especially insulin doses, food, and activity can be time-consuming and challenging. Time spent reflecting on and exploring the barriers to change can support positive behaviour change in the future.

Learning from past experience

Many people have tried to lose weight in the past, and reflecting on these experiences and exploring the advantages and disadvantages of different approaches can help with decisions about the future. Research has shown that people who successfully lose weight and, more importantly, are able to maintain that weight loss are not people who stick rigidly to one diet or another, but are people who are able to take elements from different approaches and fit them into their lifestyle. Choosing an approach that suits the individual can improve success rates.

◆ Think about your attempts at weight loss in the past—make a list of the different approaches you have used, or the different diets you have tried.

◆ Think about the advantages and disadvantages of the attempts you have made in the past. What worked and what didn't?

◆ What would you like to try now?

> ### ❓ FAQ
>
> **So, I've decided that I want to lose weight—what's the best way to do it? Is there an ideal diet for people with diabetes who want to lose weight?**
>
> There is no evidence that any one method of weight loss is the most effective. Evidence from research shows that as long as people find a diet and activity plan that suits them and that they are able to fit into their everyday life, they will be successful. Over the longer term, it makes sense to choose a way of eating that provides all the necessary nutrients, vitamins and minerals that are needed for health. For this reason, diets based on one food, such as the grapefruit diet, the egg diet, or the cabbage soup diet, are not recommended.

Table 2.5 Advantages and disadvantages of different weight loss approaches

Popular approach for weight loss	What is it?	Advantages	Disadvantages
Slimming clubs, e.g. WeightWatchers, Slimming World, Rosemary Conley	Usually group weekly meetings with a weigh-in and lectures or discussions about various topics. Some include exercise	◆ Group support and encouragement ◆ Advice about specific eating plans ◆ Regular meetings ◆ Offer weight maintenance programmes	◆ Can be expensive ◆ May set unrealistic target weights ◆ Little evidence for long-term effectiveness ◆ Not subject to regulation, may offer unsafe or unbalanced advice
Internet sites	Sites offering anything from individual meal plans to supplements and herbal remedies for weight loss	◆ Offer individual information, some offer support via chat rooms ◆ Easy to access for those with the internet ◆ Large choice available	◆ Usually charge a fee ◆ Only suitable for the computer-literate

(continued)

Table 2.5 Advantages and disadvantages of different weight loss approaches *(continued)*

Popular approach for weight loss	What is it?	Advantages	Disadvantages
Calorie-controlled diets	Diet sheets offering prescribed daily energy intake—usually 1200, 1500, or1800 calories	◆ Encourage regular, daily, energy-restricted food intake ◆ Encourage intake of healthy, low calorie fruit and vegetables ◆ No food is forbidden but high energy foods are restricted	◆ Can be prescriptive and inflexible ◆ Requires knowledge of energy value of food ◆ Requires some mathematical calculation
Low-fat, healthy diet	General nutritional recommendations including low fat, low sugar diet high in fruit and vegetables	◆ Relatively simple advice ◆ Nutritionally sound ◆ No food is forbidden	◆ Many people with diabetes adopt a healthy diet without weight loss ◆ Portion restriction must be addressed to facilitate weight loss
Low carbohydrate diets, e.g. Atkins, South Beach	Diets based on meat, fish, eggs and cheese, and salad and green vegetables. Starchy and sugary foods, fruit, and milk severely restricted	◆ Rapid, dramatic weight loss ◆ Immediate impact on blood glucose levels ◆ Suppresses appetite ◆ People often report a feeling of well-being on these diets	◆ Restricts intake of fruit and milk ◆ Some side effects—headache and constipation ◆ Nothing known about long-term effects
Meal replacements	A pre-prepared drink, meal or snack taken in place of two meals a day	◆ Provide simple, structured daily plan ◆ Minimizes food preparation and cooking ◆ Published studies show they work	◆ Can be expensive ◆ Limited range of foods and drinks available ◆ Need to continue with one replacement a day to maintain weight loss long term

(continued)

Table 2.5 Advantages and disadvantages of different weight loss approaches *(continued)*

Popular approach for weight loss	What is it?	Advantages	Disadvantages
Very low calorie diets	Nutritionally balanced drinks or bars used to replace all meals. Typically, no other food is taken other than additional fluids	◆ Rapid dramatic weight loss ◆ Simple to adopt ◆ Nutritionally balanced	◆ Does not address food-related issues ◆ Cannot be adopted long-term ◆ Rapid weight loss frequently accompanied by rapid weight gain
Fad diets, e.g. grapefruit diet, egg diet, cabbage soup diet	Designed to restrict energy intake by offering extremely restricted choice of food, often only one food	◆ Rapid, dramatic weight loss	◆ Not nutritionally balanced ◆ Designed for short-term use ◆ Rapid weight loss frequently accompanied by rapid weight gain

Diabetes medication

... but since I go onto the insulin, suddenly I put on a lot of weight, And now it's catch-22, that I want to reduce my weight. For a reduction in weight, I have to control my diet, eat less or something, but if I eat less, I get a hypo in the daytime or evening time, which is frightening. But if I eat, I'm not losing my weight.

Tas   type 2 diabetes

> ### ❓ FAQ
>
> **I've tried very hard to lose weight, but it's impossible because of the medication I have to take for my diabetes. Should I just give up?**
>
> It is not impossible for people with diabetes to lose weight, but some medication, especially insulin, can slow down weight loss. If you are trying to lose weight, but find that you are having hypos, you will need to adjust your medication. Discuss this with your healthcare team.

People who treat diabetes with insulin or sulphonylurea tablets may be at increased risk of hypoglycaemia if a reduction in the amount of food eaten is not accompanied by a reduction in medication. It is recommended that weight reduction takes place under medical supervision until an individual is confident with self-management.

> ### ❓ FAQ
>
> **I've been overweight all my life—I'll never reach my ideal weight so is there any point in bothering?**
>
> People with diabetes don't have to lose a huge amount of weight to feel the benefit, and studies have shown us that you don't need to reach your ideal weight to make a big difference. Just losing 5–10% of your starting weight can have an impact on your diabetes and your general health. Of course, the more weight you lose, the better your overall health will be.

Weight maintenance

> . . . I'd actually lost a stone since last January, which they were over the moon about. Well, I wasn't because I thought I should have lost two stone by then, but they said that's the best way to lose it—slowly, you know.
>
> Christina type 1 diabetes

? FAQ

Now that I've managed to lose weight, I don't want it all to go straight back on—what shall I do now?

You can guarantee that if you decide to go back to your old eating and exercise patterns, all the weight you have worked so hard to lose will go back on. Think about changes that you can make that will not compromise your lifestyle. Some studies have looked at people who have successfully lost weight and have identified the factors that are associated with successful maintenance. These factors are shown as top tips.

Top tips for weight maintenance

- Have regular meals, at regular times and avoid snacking.

- Regularly monitor what you eat, either by writing it down or by keeping a diary in your head.

- Monitor your weight regularly either by weighing or by how your clothes feel.

- Think about portion size. You needn't exclude any food from your diet, but limit the amount and frequency of high fat, high sugar foods.

- Continue with a low fat diet with plenty of fruit and vegetables.

- Try to avoid 'all or nothing' thinking—if you occasionally eat too much, try to limit the feelings of guilt and avoid eating even more.

- Try to manage stress and deal with problems rather than turning to food for comfort.

- Look for support from family and friends.

Smoking

➔ Key points

◆ Smoking doubles the risk of heart disease and stroke.

◆ Smoking is associated with increased kidney and nerve damage.

◆ Smoking is a physical and psychological addiction.

Most people know that smoking is bad for their health and that they should give up, but nicotine is one of the most addictive substances known. There are two aspects to tobacco addiction: physical and psychological. The combination of these two can make stopping smoking very challenging.

The best-known effect of smoking is that it causes lung cancer, but smoking is also associated with other aspects of diabetes, and stopping smoking can reduce risks significantly.

❓ FAQ

Why does my doctor keep going on about smoking? Surely it's no worse for me than for anyone else?

Unfortunately, smoking has been shown to be associated with premature death and much of the tissue damage seen in people with diabetes:

◆ Lung disease, cardiovascular disease, cancer, and stroke are more common in people who smoke.

◆ Kidney disease (nephropathy) is more common in people with diabetes who smoke, and for people who already have established kidney disease, non-smokers do better than smokers.

◆ Nerve damage (neuropathy) develops more frequently and progresses more rapidly in smokers than in non-smokers.

Top tips for stopping smoking

- Find a temporary replacement habit such as chewing gum. Try not to use food as a replacement for cigarettes if you are worried about weight gain.

- Change your routine to avoid places, situations, or people you associate with smoking.

- Pick a suitable date to stop smoking—and stick to it!

- Don't try cutting down—stop completely.

- Find support from friends and family. Ask your healthcare professional if there is a local group you could join for support.

- Keep trying—most smokers can't give up the first time they try.

Now, obviously, like most people you don't just decide (to stop) smoking, you have several goes. (My wife) she decided to stop as well. So, you know, there was support for either of us, from each other and we managed it eventually.

Hans   type 1 diabetes

I smoked a pipe until my mid-thirties, when under pressure from my wife who had given up six months before, I finally managed to get it together and give up smoking. Within a year of that, she even started smoking again, but I managed to stay off the weed and I haven't smoked since.

Peter   type 1 diabetes

Being a healthcare professional—definitely I would advise anyone to give up smoking, and I would advise myself to give up smoking, I guess, but I'm not quite there yet—but don't start; give it up

Mary   type 1 diabetes

Methods for stopping smoking

Many people quote will-power as the best way to give up smoking, and this seems to be required to some degree whatever method is used, but will-power alone is not as effective as using it in combination with other treatments. Using nicotine replacement therapy or medication can double chances of success; these in combination with group sessions or behavioural therapy can increase the likelihood of stopping smoking fourfold.

But then, at one time, I decided 'ugh'—it was enough; I'd had enough. And it was a waste of money really, and I didn't really enjoy it, so I just decided to give up smoking. I didn't have any withdrawal symptoms or anything, so I gave up on that day and never smoked again.

Edward   type 2 diabetes

Table 2.6 Advantages and disadvantages of different approaches to stopping smoking

Approach	Description	Advantages	Disadvantages
Cold turkey	Stopping smoking suddenly relying on will-power	• Cheap • Least complicated method • Safe • No side effects from nicotine	• Least effective method • Less likely to stay smoke-free than by using nicotine replacement or medication
Nicotine replacement therapy (NRT)	Provides nicotine to relieve physical symptoms of addiction without smoking cigarettes	• Using NRT doubles chance of success	• People with diabetes should discuss use of NRT with their doctor—it may not be suitable for all
Examples: Nicotine gum	Supplies nicotine from chewing gum when needed	• Simple to use • Few side effects • Breaks smoking habit	• May dislike chewing in public • Unpleasant taste • Small risk of mouth ulcers, indigestion or jaw pain

(continued)

Table 2.6 Advantages and disadvantages of different approaches to stopping smoking (*continued*)

Approach	Description	Advantages	Disadvantages
Nicotine patches	Supply small, constant s dose of nicotine over 16–24 hours	• Simple to use • Discrete • Different strengths for different people	• Skin irritation or rashes • Only effective for 8 weeks • Easy to smoke while using patches
Nicotine inhalator	Cigarette-shaped inhaler delivering nicotine when needed	• Simple to use • Provides physical substitute for cigarettes	• Can cause sore mouth • Some dislike taste • Reinforces dependence on cigarettes
Medication:			
Bupropion (Zyban)	Acts in the brain to reduce cravings for cigarettes and nicotine. Available as 8 week course	• Doubles the chance of success • Reduces the urge to smoke • Reduces withdrawal symptoms	• Only available on prescription • Side effects include dry mouth, insomnia, headaches and appetite change • Rarely causes seizures
Varenicline	Centrally acting drug reducing craving and withdrawal symptoms. Available as 12 week course	• Trebles the chance of success • Reduces cravings and withdrawal	• Only available on prescription • Main side effect is nausea
Alternative therapies e.g. hypnosis, acupuncture	Therapies designed to reduce cravings and withdrawal, and support will-power	• Many people feel these therapies provide much-needed support	• No evidence that they are effective • Can be expensive

Alcohol

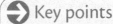 **Key points**

- Alcohol can be drunk in moderation by most people with diabetes.

- General safe drinking recommendations apply.

- People taking insulin or sulphonylureas are at increased risk of hypoglycaemia after alcohol.

- Large amounts of sugary drinks will raise blood glucose levels.

- Pregnant women should avoid alcohol.

DON'T DRINK AND DRIVE

Alcohol in moderate amounts can be enjoyed safely by people with diabetes. The general advice about alcohol use is the same as for people without diabetes, but there are some aspects that need consideration. Some people with diabetes may be advised not to drink alcohol for health reasons.

? FAQ

Is it safe for me to drink alcohol if I have diabetes?

Most people with diabetes can drink alcohol safely, but there are a few exceptions:

- If you have ever been told that you have high triglycerides (a fat in the blood) or high blood pressure, then drinking alcohol can raise your levels further.

- If you have nerve damage (neuropathy) then alcohol can increase the pain and make the condition worse.

- Heavy, regular drinking (more than 3–4 units daily) can make the eye condition known as retinopathy worse.

- If you have diabetes and are pregnant, alcohol should be avoided.

Effect of alcohol in the body

Alcohol is treated as a poison by the body and is broken down (metabolized) by the liver. The liver has many functions in the body, one of which is to release stored glucose into the bloodstream when blood glucose levels start to drop. This helps prevent hypoglycaemia (low blood glucose levels). After alcohol, the liver is employed with clearing the alcohol and if blood glucose levels drop, the liver will not produce glucose to help raise levels again. This increases the risk of hypoglycaemia, especially in people who take insulin or sulphonylurea tablets to treat diabetes. This hypoglycaemic effect of alcohol can last up to 24 hours after a drinking session.

Tips for avoiding hypoglycaemia

◆ Try to avoid drinking on an empty stomach.

◆ Eat some starchy carbohydrate foods before or with alcoholic drinks. You may need a snack before bed after drinking alcohol in the evening.

◆ Keep to sensible drinking levels—large amounts of alcohol will increase the risk of hypos.

◆ Keep some fast-acting carbohydrate with you to treat hypoglycaemic symptoms as soon as they occur. Remember that the early signs of hypos may be confused with the effects of alcohol.

❓ FAQ

I keep hearing about safe drinking—what does this mean?

Many governments publish safe drinking advice for people whether they have diabetes or not. This advice varies from country to country. In the UK the advice can be summarized as follows:

◆ Men can drink up to 3–4 units each day and women 2–3 units daily. Recommendations used to be made over the week (men's allowance was 21–28 units and women's 14–21 units weekly, but some people saved their weekly allowance up and had them all in one night— known as binge drinking).

- Binge drinking causes severe health and social problems and should be avoided.

- Have 2–3 days each week when you don't drink at all.

What's a unit?

The amount of alcohol differs in different drinks. These days, many drinks (especially strong beers and wine) contain more alcohol than formerly and it is easy to have the full daily allowance in just one drink. For example, sharing a standard 750 ml bottle of 13% wine would give two people 5 units of alcohol each.

A pint of ordinary strength lager = 2 units

A pint of strong lager = 3 units

A pint of bitter = 2 units

A pint of ordinary strength cider = 2 units

A 175 ml glass of red or white wine = 2 units (approximately)

A pub measure of spirits = 1 unit

An alcopop = 1.5 units (approximately)

A can of beer or lager = 1.5 units

Carbohydrate content of drinks

The amount of carbohydrate in alcohol can vary greatly. Some alcoholic drinks contain little or no carbohydrate (dry wines, spirits), some contain moderate amounts (beer, lager, cider) and some contain significant amounts (alcopops, sweet sherry and wines, port). The effect of alcoholic drinks on blood glucose levels will depend upon the amount and the type of alcohol drunk. Large amounts of sweet drinks can raise blood glucose levels significantly, and this can be minimized by:

- Using diet soft drinks, soda, or water as mixers with spirits.

- Choosing light beer or lager or a dry wine.

- Alternating alcoholic drinks with diet drinks, soda, or mineral water.

Alcohol and weight control

Moderate drinking may not affect blood glucose control, but some alcoholic drinks are high in calories and can sabotage weight loss. Alcohol is often described as containing 'empty calories' as it provides calories but few other useful vitamins and minerals. Individuals who wish to lose weight are advised to limit or avoid alcoholic drinks as this can slow down or stop planned weight loss.

Recreational drugs

➜ Key points

- Most recreational drugs are illegal.

- Recreational drug use may be associated with physical or psychological addiction and mental and physical health problems.

- People with diabetes may find that using recreational drugs can interfere with the usual routines of blood glucose testing, medication, and regular meals.

I used to drink Martini Bianco, I remember that, but I didn't do drugs at all. I thought, I've got enough drugs going into my body.

Patsy   type 1 diabetes

There were things I didn't do, because I was diabetic. I didn't really understand how LSD worked, but I knew it worked on your sugars and I didn't want to have a bad time. But I did meet someone who I thought was very silly towards his diabetes, because he used to do all sorts of drugs and say 'Oh, I will just make sure my sugars are really high before I take them, so I wouldn't have a hypo'.

Clare   type 1 diabetes

Most recreational drugs are illegal, but in the cultural climate among young people today it is inevitable that some people will experiment with recreational drugs. People with diabetes who choose to take drugs should be aware of the impact this may have on their diabetes care and the potential risks to their health.

Table 2.7 The effects of various recreational drugs

Drug	Action	Effect on diabetes	General side effects
Stimulants (uppers):	Speed up metabolism	Can cause hypos—often hypo symptoms can be overlooked	Intense high is followed by extended low
Cocaine (coke), crack	Produce a brief, intense high Make the heart beat harder	Have an effect on blood glucose levels Can cause problems with heart function	Highly addictive Can affect personality and induce paranoia
Amphetamines (speed)	Increases energy Induces wakefulness Depresses appetite	Increased energy expenditure and appetite suppression lead to hypos	Used regularly, side effects are similar to cocaine
Ecstasy (e)	Induces a feel-good factor	Can cause dehydration and hypos—especially if used while clubbing	Can affect personality
Depressants (downers): Heroin	Slows down heart rate, speed of thinking Induces feeling of calm	Interferes with normal routines of diabetes care Can disrupt usual hypo symptoms	Addictive Injecting carries the risk of HIV and hepatitis Overdosing leads to coma and death
Tranquillizers	Relieve anxiety Induce feeling of calm	Short-term memory loss and sleepiness Can disrupt usual routines of diabetes care	Addictive Can cause coma Risk of overdose, especially if used with alcohol
Hallucinogens:	Alter perceptions—including sight, hearing, and feelings	Losing track of time affects usual diabetes care	Heavy users may develop mental health problems such as psychosis
Cannabis (dope, weed, blow)	Induces a high	Stimulates appetite—the 'munchies'—which may lead to overeating	Panic attacks Long-term mental health problems

(continued)

Table 2.7 The effects of various recreational drugs *(continued)*

Drug	Action	Effect on diabetes	General side effects
LSD and magic mushrooms	Induces hallucinations known as a 'trip'	Loss of sense of time interferes with usual routines May alter perception of hypos	Bad trips cause physical and psychological distress Flash backs Some mushrooms are poisonous
Solvents	Produce an immediate high	Forgetfulness may lead to missed medication Over time, may damage liver and kidneys	Headache May trigger violent or unpredictable behaviour Long-term health problems Death

3

Medication

Oral medication and diabetes

→ Key points

- There are five types of oral medication available: metformin, sulphonylureas, glitazones, acarbose, and meglitinides.

- The most commonly prescribed first-line medications are metformin, which acts to enhance the effects of insulin, and sulphonylureas, which increase insulin secretion.

- The main side effects of metformin are nausea and diarrhoea, but these do improve with time and can be reduced by increasing the dose gradually.

- The main side effect of sulphonylureas is hypoglycaemia.

- Glitazones are useful if metformin is not tolerated or as a third medication to add to metformin and a sulphonylurea if the blood sugars are not controlled.

- Acarbose and the meglitinides are useful for controlling post-meal rises in glucose.

- There are currently three drugs available to aid weight loss, but these must be used in conjunction with diet and exercise.

- The majority of people with type 2 diabetes will also require cardiovascular medications (statins, aspirin, and blood pressure tablets)— see Chapter 5.

It is an exciting time in the treatment history of diabetes: there has been much development firstly in the types of oral medications available and secondly in the forms of insulin available, as well as the different ways to administer it.

> ### 'I want to take pills for my diabetes. I don't want to take insulin'
>
> As yet, the oral agents available cannot take the place of insulin. All the tablets that are used for diabetes require a person to be making at least some insulin from his or her own pancreas. Insulin itself cannot be given by mouth as it is a fragile chemical that is immediately destroyed by the stomach acids if given orally. Thus the bottom line is that oral medications will not work if a person has type 1 diabetes: they will have to rely on insulin injections. Also, tablets often do not work when type 2 diabetes has progressed to the point where the person is secreting very little insulin from the pancreas. Type 2 diabetes is characterized by a progressive loss of the insulin-producing beta-cells in the pancreas such that around 50% of people with type 2 diabetes will need insulin within 5 years of diagnosis.

The main treatment in type 2 diabetes is with oral medications, although insulin can be added later: the main treatment in type 1 diabetes is with insulin.

Although diet and lifestyle changes remain the first-line treatments for type 2 diabetes, most people (80–90%) will require some form of medication to achieve good long-term control and reduce the chance of complications. Importantly, tablets are only truly effective if used in conjunction with a healthy diet and regular exercise.

Oral medications

Tablets are not useful in treating type 1 diabetes or in gestational diabetes because of possible injury to the developing foetus. Occasionally, when it is not clear if the correct diagnosis is type 1 or type 2 diabetes, tablets may be given a trial use. The drug types available all have different actions: which drug is recommended will therefore depend on the particular features of a person's diabetes. In most cases insulin resistance (a lower effect of insulin) is a major problem and therefore metformin is often the first drug recommended.

I have to admit I don't always remember to take my tablets . . .

The oral medications are most effective if taken regularly every day, and not started and stopped according to blood glucose. They work best to maintain a steady blood glucose and are not meant to be taken just when the blood glucose is already too high or if a person is feeling unwell. Therefore they should not be stopped just on a whim. If one is worried about an allergic reaction (typically characterized by a widespread rash, hives, or difficulty breathing), they can of course be stopped and alternative medications discussed with a healthcare professional. Specific possible side effects are discussed below.

Glucose-lowering therapies for type 2 diabetes

There are five main types of tablet that are now used to treat type 2 diabetes:

◆ Metformin

◆ Sulphonylureas

◆ Acarbose

◆ Thiazolidinediones (glitazones)

◆ Meglitinides

Table 3.1 summarizes some features of each type of medication, which are then discussed in more detail.

Table 3.1 Features of each type of glucose-lowering medication

Drug	Brand names	Action	Dosage	Side effects
Metformin	Glucophage	Increases effect of insulin on the body's tissues	500–2500 mg daily with food	Nausea, diarrhoea
Extended release metformin	Glucophage XR		500–2000 mg daily	
Sulphonylureas:		Stimulate insulin secretion by the pancreas		Hypoglycaemia
Gliclazide	Diamicron		40–160 mg twice daily	
Extended release gliclazide	Diamicron MR		30–120 mg daily	
Glibenclamide	Daonil/Euglucon		5–15 mg daily	
Glipizide	Glibenese/ Minodab		2.5–20 mg twice daily	
Glimepiride	Amaryl		1–4 mg once daily	

(continued)

Table 3.1 Features of each type of glucose-lowering medication *(continued)*

Drug	Brand names	Action	Dosage	Side effects
Acarbose	Glucobay	Slows absorption of carbohydrate from intestine	50–100 mg three times daily with food	Diarrhoea, wind, bloating
Glitazones:		Enhance action of insulin		Weight gain Fluid retention
Rosiglitazone	Avandia		4–8 mg daily	
Pioglitazone	Actos		15–45 mg daily	
Meglitinides:	Increase insulin secretion after food			Hypoglycaemia
Repaglinide	Prandin		2 mg	
Nateglinide	Starlix		60–120 mg twice daily before meals	

Metformin

Metformin is the most commonly prescribed drug for diabetes and has been used in the UK since the 1970s. It is derived from guanidine, an active ingredient found in French lilac. This plant was one of the earliest traditional remedies for diabetes in Europe. It is recommended as first-line treatment in type 2 diabetes and is particularly useful as it does not cause weight gain and can actually help weight loss by its gastrointestinal side effects. Recently it has become available in a once daily/slow release preparation which is reported to cause fewer side effects and is also a good option for those often forgetting to take their medication. Around 10% of patients do not respond to metformin, and approximately 5–10% patients a year on metformin will need another agent in addition.

Action

Metformin's mechanism of action is unclear, but it appears to act at three sites:

- It increases the effect of insulin in the body's tissues (especially muscle), causing more efficient uptake and use of blood glucose.

- It helps suppress excess glucose production by the liver.

- It is also thought to slow the uptake of glucose from the gut.

In this way metformin can also aid the action of insulin given by injection and therefore be considered a supplement to sulphonylureas or insulin therapy.

Metformin is excreted unchanged by the kidneys.

Side effects

These may occur in up to 30% of people taking metformin, and the most well-recognized adverse effects are:

◆ Nausea, abdominal discomfort, or diarrhoea. Gastrointestinal side effects are the most common side effect of metformin. It is less of a problem if the dose started is small and increased gradually, and usually this side effect goes away with time.

◆ Weight loss. This may be due to the above side effect or because it can make food have less taste.

◆ Reduced vitamin B12 absorption. Vitamin B12 is required for the blood and the nervous system, and occasionally metformin causes a decrease in its absorption from the intestine.

◆ Lactic acidosis. This is a very rare complication but is the reason why metformin is not given to people who have impaired kidney function.

Metformin does not cause hypoglycaemia itself as it does not directly increase insulin secretion. However, this can occur if given in combination with a sulphonylurea.

People with the following should not take metformin:

◆ Impaired kidney function

◆ Pregnant women or breastfeeding mothers

◆ Significant liver disease

◆ Heart failure

◆ History of alcohol abuse

◆ People undergoing a specialized X-ray that requires injection of a dye or people having surgery should omit metformin for 24–48 hours beforehand.

Sulphonylureas

Sulphonylureas were discovered by chance during the Second World War when it was noticed that soldiers treated with sulphonamide antibiotics experienced a drop in blood glucose. They have been used for over 50 years and there are now the so-called second-generation sulphonylureas available, noted in Table 3.1, which were developed in the 1970s and 1980s. They are taken at much lower doses than the earlier sulphonylureas but act in a similar way. For those liable to forget to take the tablets twice daily, there are now slow release preparations that can be taken once daily such as glimepiride (Amaryl) and glipizide (Glucotrol XL). The newer sulphonylureas are also less likely to have interactions with other medications a person may be taking. Essentially all the different sulphonylureas act by the same basic mechanisms, share some side effects and it is unlikely that if a person fails to respond to one sulphonylurea they will respond to another.

Action

All sulphonylureas share the same basic mechanisms:

◆ They stimulate insulin secretion from the pancreas by enhancing its reaction to blood glucose levels.

◆ If the pancreas is too weak to make much insulin, they are not effective. Therefore, even if they work for a while, these tablets may not be effective permanently, as the pancreas tends to produce less insulin over years.

◆ They help the pancreas to secrete this insulin throughout the day and night as well as in response to meals.

◆ They are inactivated by the liver and excreted by the kidneys.

❓ FAQ

I initially had awful hypos on sulphonylureas, is there a way to avoid this?

Whichever sulphonylurea is prescribed, it should be started at a low dose and the blood sugar should be checked regularly. This is then increased every 2–4 weeks until the blood sugar is adequately controlled.

If on starting a sulphonylurea a person develops symptoms of hypoglycaemia which are confirmed by a blood sugar reading during one of these episodes, a doctor may reduce the dose or change to a different sulphonylurea.

Long-acting sulphonylureas such as glibenclamide are associated with higher risk of hypoglycaemia and should be avoided in elderly patients.

Regular meals can reduce risk of hypoglycaemia. Drinking excess alcohol while on a sulphonylurea also increases the risk of hypoglycaemia.

Side effects

Common side effects are:

* Hypoglycaemia

* Weight gain of approximately 1–4 kg in the first 6 months (about 3 kg on average)

Uncommon side effects include:

* Rash

* Headache, diarrhoea, wind

As with metformin, pregnant women and breastfeeding mothers should not take sulphonylureas.

Acarbose

Acarbose (Glucobay) is one of the so-called alpha-glucosidase inhibitors and has been around since the 1990s. It reduces the after-meal rise in blood sugar and brings about a modest reduction in haemoglobin A1c (HbA1c) compared with other oral agents. It is only effective in those with adequate insulin production and should therefore be used early in the course of type 2 diabetes.

Action

* Acarbose acts by blocking the enzymes in the intestine that break down the long chains of glucose in starch and sugar into their component smaller molecules of glucose in order to be absorbed.

* The effect of blocking this breakdown is to slow the absorption of carbohydrate after a meal. This carbohydrate goes on to be broken down lower in the intestine.

* The drug itself is not absorbed into the blood but acts locally, in the intestine.

To be effective, it should be taken with the first mouthful of food. The starting dose is usually 50 mg once a day, which can be increased up to 100 mg three times a day.

Side effects

Acarbose causes increased gas production in as many as 75% of users and is the major disadvantage of this drug. The most common side effects are:

◆ Wind, abdominal pain, bloating, and diarrhoea. This can be reduced by starting at a low dose and building up gradually.

◆ Acarbose itself does not cause hypoglycaemia. If hypoglycaemia caused by other agents occurs, then this should be treated by pure glucose (either dextrose tablets or Lucozade).

People with the following should not take acarbose:

◆ Inflammatory bowel disease such as ulcerative colitis or Crohn's disease

◆ Hernia

◆ History of abdominal surgery

◆ Liver failure

◆ Kidney failure

◆ Pregnant women or breastfeeding mothers

Thiazolidinediones

This group of drugs (also known as the 'glitazones') have been used only relatively recently, since 1997. The first glitazone used, troglitazone, was withdrawn in 2000 because of an association with liver damage. This drug has been superseded by rosiglitazone (Avandia) and pioglitazone (Actos), neither of which have been linked to liver damage. They are taken once daily, starting with a low dose, and take for up to 3 months to have their maximum effect. They produce a lowering of blood glucose levels comparable to being on metformin or a sulphonylurea alone.

Action

- The glitazones act to make the body's tissues more sensitive to insulin.

- Therefore, a person does not have to produce as much insulin to control blood glucose when they are taking a glitazone.

- Glitazones tend to be given as second- or third-line therapy, partly because of the 10–12 weeks it takes for them to have an effect. Generally a person is offered a combination of metformin and a sulphonylurea before a glitazone is added in. Glitazones are also often prescribed if a person cannot tolerate metformin. They are inactivated in the liver and excreted either in urine or in bile from the liver.

'Triple therapy'

If the blood glucose is still not controlled sufficiently with metformin and a sulphonylurea, a trial of 'triple therapy', i.e. with metformin, a sulphonylurea and a glitazone, can be an alternative to starting insulin.

Side effects

- Weight gain of 1–4 kg in the first 6–12 months.

- Fluid retention.

- Anaemia because of the extra fluid retained.

- Women who have reduced fertility because of insulin resistance may find their fertility improves on a glitazone and they may become pregnant (in which case the drug should be stopped).

- In themselves they do not cause hypos.

People with the following should not take a glitazone:

- Liver disease

- Heart failure

> - Leg oedema
>
> - Anaemia
>
> - Pregnant women or breastfeeding mothers

Although neither rosiglitazone nor pioglitazone have been linked to liver damage, it is recommended that a person's liver function tests are checked when starting the drug and repeated a couple of months after having been on the drug.

Meglitinides

Meglitinides, such as repaglinide (Prandin) and netaglinide (Starlix), are short-acting agents that are used to control post-meal (or postprandial) rises in glucose. They are taken up to 30 minutes before main meals and stimulate insulin for that meal, i.e. they have no effect in between meals.

Action

- Meglitinides stimulate insulin secretion from the pancreas.

- They are rapidly absorbed from the intestine and then completely inactivated by the liver in less than an hour. This means the drug causes a brief but rapid surge of insulin appropriate for postprandial rises in blood glucose.

Side effects

- Hypoglycaemia

- Abdominal pain, diarrhoea, constipation, nausea, vomiting

- Weight gain

- Rash

Pregnant women or breastfeeding mothers should not take meglitinides. They are also not recommended in those with severe liver disease or people who are under 18 or over 75.

Weight loss medications

These are a useful adjunct to the oral medications for type 2 diabetes. Of course diet and exercise are the crucial elements in any weight loss plan, but in those who are well motivated there are some medications available to help. As being overweight is such a contributory factor to type 2 diabetes, weight loss drugs, if taken consistently with a healthy lifestyle, can cause significant reduction in HbA1c and blood glucose levels, as well as blood pressure and cholesterol. There are three main drugs currently available:

Orlistat (Xenical)

◆ Acts by reducing absorption of fat from the gut.

◆ The fat stays in the intestine and stool, and therefore the main side effect is gas and oily bowel movements.

◆ It is given if a person's BMI is over 28 and they have type 2 diabetes, and have lost at least 5 lb with diet and exercise alone in the month before starting the drug.

◆ It is usually only prescribed for 1–2 years and only continues if there is 10% weight loss in the first 6 months.

Sibutramine (Reductil)

◆ Acts by reducing re-uptake of particular hormones (serotonin and noradrenaline) to make people feel full sooner and therefore eat smaller portions of food.

◆ It can cause an increase in blood pressure and heart rate, and therefore is only given to people whose blood pressure is below 145/90 mmHg. If on starting the drug the blood pressure rises by more than 10 mmHg the medication is stopped.

◆ It is available if a person's BMI is over 28 and they have type 2 diabetes.

◆ It will continue to be prescribed if there is 5% weight loss in the first 3 months and it can be continued for 1 year.

Rimonabant

◆ Acts by blocking the cannabinoid-1 receptor. This is one of the receptors used by cannabis which is an appetite stimulant. Therefore, it makes sense that by blocking it weight loss may be enhanced.

◆ Side effects include nausea, diarrhoea, dizziness, anxiety, and insomnia.

- It should not be taken if a person suffers with severe depression or is taking antidepressants.

- Has been used in many drug trials with largely favourable results not only on weight loss but also in reducing HbA1c and cholesterol.

Each drug is only useful if the person is committed to reducing weight with diet and exercise. The medication can help as part of a general lifestyle change and should be taken with advice from a dietician.

Insulin

→ Key points

- Insulin is crucial in type 1 diabetes and is recommended in up to 50% of people with type 2 diabetes within 5 years.

- Human insulin is now the main form of insulin used as opposed to animal insulin.

- There are several forms of insulin available with varying durations of action.

- People with type 1 diabetes can be on twice-daily insulin, but a more intensive regime with basal–bolus therapy is usually recommended for optimum control and prevention of complications.

- It is most common to start people with type 2 diabetes on one injection of long-acting insulin at bedtime.

- Insulin pens are now the most common mode of delivery and have been designed for ease and comfort of use.

Insulin is life saving in people with type 1 diabetes and a crucial addition to treatment in people with type 2 diabetes who reach the stage when their own pancreas is not making enough. Technological advances have meant it is now available in very pure forms that, if given correctly, can closely resemble the body's normal insulin response. Although being on insulin still inevitably means giving injections, easier and more comfortable methods have been developed which hopefully make the practicalities less daunting.

How insulin works

When someone has been suffering from a lack of insulin they usually feel a huge difference on starting insulin therapy, especially those who have been diagnosed with type 1 diabetes: it relieves the insatiable thirst and constant urination (by lowering blood glucose); it returns body strength (by promoting muscle development); and it allows the regain of normal fat stores (by promoting the storage of calories as fat).

1. Lowering blood glucose

   Blood glucose comes from the diet, but also the liver which makes 'new glucose' from storage forms of glucose (glycogen) or from protein. Insulin lowers blood sugar by both increasing the removal of glucose from the blood and reducing the production of glucose by the liver. Insulin makes the body's cells take up glucose as a source of energy.

2. Building muscle

   Insulin helps the delivery of the building blocks of muscle protein, amino acids, to the muscles.

3. Fat storage

   This may sound unappealing but we all need a certain amount of extra calories stored as fat and glycogen so that they can be used by the body in unpredicted fasts. Insulin promotes this storage.

Making the decision to take insulin

> **?** FAQ
>
> ### Does starting insulin mean my diabetes is worse?
>
> To a certain extent it is, as the requirement for insulin means the pancreas is increasingly unable to do the job despite lifestyle changes and tablets. However, it is the prevention of complications that is pivotal in order to maintain well-being, and if insulin is required to keep severe complications at bay, then most people would choose to take it.
>
> ### Will I need insulin forever?
>
> Most often yes, but not always. In type 2 diabetes, weight loss and exercise improve the body's response to insulin. This can lead to reducing the insulin dose and in some people stopping it altogether. People with type 1 diabetes will almost certainly need insulin 'forever'.

> I feel so much better since I've been on the insulin . . . I wish I had started taking it sooner.

Some people are reluctant to go on to insulin but appreciate its need with a dramatic improvement in their symptoms and energy levels. Although it can seem unimaginable to incorporate a series of injections into the daily routine (particularly for those just diagnosed with type 1 diabetes), virtually everyone quickly takes it in their stride. If a person's healthcare provider recommends insulin, while it is worthwhile concentrating on some improvements that may make a difference; procrastinating for months will only lead to increased chance of complications. Therefore, it is good to set a target date, say 1 or 2 months, for the blood glucose to come down. Committing to insulin use does not have to mean a complete upheaval in lifestyle.

Some key principles of insulin use

- ◆ The choice of insulin regime and dose depends on several factors: what type of diabetes a person has; their weight; their age; how much they check or intend to check their blood glucose; and finally, what goals they are trying to achieve.

- ◆ The principle of insulin replacement is to mimic insulin secretion in a person without diabetes. After eating, there is normally a rapid rise in insulin to limit glucose levels after meals. Overnight low, steady levels of insulin (the background or 'basal' insulin) are sufficient to limit glucose production by the liver.

Type 1 principles

◆ In type 1 diabetes there is almost no insulin left in the pancreas, therefore requiring a more comprehensive insulin regime that can be fine-tuned. People will start on at least two injections a day and potentially increase to four injections reasonably quickly to give more control.

◆ There is no universal recommendation for what dose to start on. However, a daily dose of 16–24 units is appropriate for the majority of adult patients. A person can be started on a much lower or higher dose than this depending on their weight.

◆ Many people with type 1 diabetes have a 'honeymoon' period on starting insulin when their pancreas appears to recover. It can start within a month and last up to a year. The need for insulin can drop dramatically and it is thought the remaining insulin-producing cells of the pancreas have a period of increased activity when there is now other insulin available.

Type 2 principles

◆ In type 2 diabetes the pancreas does still make some insulin, but the injected insulin is intended to take the pressure off the reserves which are left in the body. The doses generally are not as complex, and often just one or two injections a day are enough.

◆ Usually the amount of insulin required is higher in type 2 diabetes (often 50–150 units a day, especially for larger people). This high requirement is not related to how 'bad' the diabetes is; rather, it is a reflection of how sensitive the body is to insulin.

Table 3.2 Types of insulin

Type	Name	Onset	Peak	Length of action
Short-acting analogue	Insulin aspart (Novorapid) Insulin lispro (Humalog) Insulin glulisine (Apidra)	5 minutes	1 hour	3 hours
Short-acting soluble	Actrapid (human or pork)	15–30 minutes	3 hours	6 hours

(continued)

Table 3.2 Types of insulin (*continued*)

Type	Name	Onset	Peak	Length of action
Intermediate-acting	Isophane (insulatard— human or pork, Humulin I)	1 hour	6 hours	12–18 hours
Long-acting	Detemir (Levemir) Glargine (Lantus)	1–2 hours	No real peak	12–18 hours 18–24 hours
Pre-mixed	Novomix 30, Humalog Mix 25 or 50, Mixtard 10, 20, 30, 40 or 50, Humulin M3	30 min	2–6 hours	8–12 hours

The aim of insulin treatment is to achieve the best possible control of blood glucose without causing significant hypoglycaemia. Appropriate combinations of the above insulins can be tailored to the individual: a certain element of this will be trial and error, but liaising closely with the healthcare provider eventually often results in the right regime for that person. The pre-mixed insulins are a popular starting regime, and the timing of onset, peak and duration of action will depend on the component parts.

Insulin can be kept at room temperature for 4 weeks but should then be discarded. It can be kept in the fridge until the expiration date. It should not be exposed to extremes of temperature.

Insulin injection sites

◆ The recommended sites for insulin injection are shown in Figure 3.1. Injection should be given into a pinched-up skin fold using thumb, index, and middle finger, taking up the skin and leaving the muscle behind. This will avoid intramuscular injection.

◆ Insulin absorption is fastest in the abdomen and slowest in the arms and buttocks. Short-acting insulin is best given into the abdomen, and long-acting insulin into the thigh or arm; however, this can be varied according to the most practical available site.

◆ Most importantly the injection sites should be 'rotated', i.e. if the abdomen is most often used then rotating around different points regularly is a good idea. This is to avoid lipohypertrophy (an accumulation of fat under the skin) which occurs if the same injection site is repeatedly used. If this occurs it can be unsightly and increases the variability of insulin absorption.

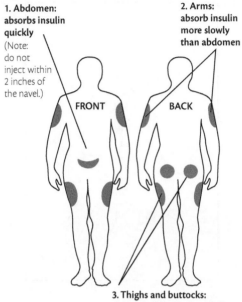

1. Abdomen: absorbs insulin quickly
(Note: do not inject within 2 inches of the navel.)

FRONT

2. Arms: absorb insulin more slowly than abdomen

BACK

3. Thighs and buttocks: absorb insulin slowest of all

Figure 3.1 Insulin injection sites.

- If a person rotates from limb to limb, it is a good idea to try and stick to a schedule whereby the same area is injected at the same time of day, e.g. morning injection in the abdomen, tea time injection in the leg.

- Insulin absorption can also be accelerated by exercising that part of the body.

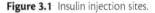

IMPORTANT: DO NOT MIX SITE AND TIME

Different insulin delivery systems

There are four main devices for insulin injection: needle and syringe; insulin pens (now most commonly used); jet injection devices; and external pumps.

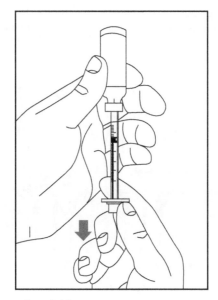

Figure 3.2 Insulin needle and vial.

Needle and syringe

This is the traditional method of delivery. The following steps are recommended:

1. Clean the rubber stopper of the bottle with alcohol. If intermediate-acting or long-acting insulin is being used (cloudy insulins), mix them by rolling or rotating the bottle.

2. Open the syringe to the number of units that is needed so that there is air to this point in the syringe.

3. Turn the insulin bottle upside down and inject the stopper with the needle.

4. Push the air inside and withdraw the insulin dose required.

5. Give the syringe a few taps with your finger to get the bubbles to the top, and push the bubbles back into the bottle.

6. Pinch up the area of skin to be injected.

7. Insert the needle at a right angle to the skin and push it in, then push down the plunger to administer the insulin.

There are now several aids to needle and syringe delivery: spring-loaded syringe holders; syringe magnifiers to help the visually impaired; syringe-filling devices which click when the insulin has been taken up; and needle guides if a person cannot see the rubber stop on the bottle where the needle is inserted to take up insulin.

Insulin pens

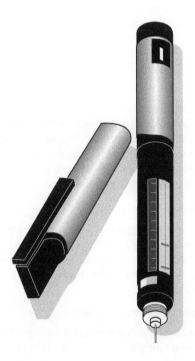

Figure 3.3 Insulin pen and needles.

These pens come with a cartridge already inserted which contains 3.0 ml of the specific insulin, and a person can dial the amount of insulin to be taken. Each unit (or two units) is accompanied by a click so that people with visual impairment can hear the number of units: the number will also appear in a window on the pen. The pens allow delivery of 30–70 units; a new needle can be screwed on as necessary. There are several different pens available and it is best to view them and try them out with a diabetes specialist nurse to see which is most suitable.

Needle issues

◆ Your practice or local authority may provide a sharps bin designed for safe disposal of needles and syringes. See Diabetes UK guidelines on disposal of sharps.

◆ 8 mm needles are most often used, but thinner people may need 5 or 6 mm to avoid intramuscular injection. This can be decided upon with the healthcare provider.

Jet injection device

These are expensive but good for people who cannot perform the injection for themselves. The device holds a large quantity of insulin to be used for multiple treatments. After dialling up the amount of insulin to be delivered, the device is held against the skin, and on pressing a button a jet of air forces the insulin through the skin into the tissue underneath. This device is occasionally leaky, with insulin staying above the skin; others report that the injection can be painful.

External insulin pumps

These are about the size of a pager and are worn on the belt or in the clothing, with thin plastic tubing coming from the pump to a needle that penetrates the skin, usually in the abdomen. It is in place 24 hours a day and this device is as close as one can get to the constant gradual administration of insulin that is taking place in the body.

Some important points to know about pumps

◆ They do not measure blood sugar and so the pump still needs to be directed by blood sugar measurements with a meter and dose adjustments.

◆ There are two basic rates of delivery: *the basal rate*, which is a slow, continuous trickle when a person is not eating; and the *bolus rate*, which is a much higher flow rate and delivered when a meal is about to be eaten.

◆ Much guidance is required, especially at the start, from the diabetes nurse and/or doctor, in addition to a dietician.

◆ NICE guidelines recommend that pumps are considered in those where other insulin regimes have 'failed'—i.e. it is impossible to reduce HbA1c to less than 7.5% without causing 'disabling hypoglycaemia'. Pumps should also only be used for people who are committed to gaining the considerable expertise and competence that the effective use of a pump requires.

Advantages of pumps

- They are flexible and good for people whose meal times are unpredictable.

- They have built-in safety devices to stop overdosage.

- They generally do improve control, reducing uncomfortable swings in blood sugar, and result in a better HbA1c.

Disadvantages of pumps

- Skin infections can occur as the infusion set is left *in situ* for a few days.

- Ketoacidosis can occur rapidly if the pump disconnects as short-acting insulin is the only form given.

- Blood glucose must be measured frequently to adjust the pump for best control.

- They are expensive (more than £2500, with annual costs of about £1200).

- Limited availability of pumps supplied from the NHS.

Inhaled insulin

A number of drug companies have developed inhaled insulins. In principle, this was a way of avoiding giving insulin by injection, but the dose of insulin needed was about seven times the amount needed compared with injection. The accuracy of dosing proved difficult and because the insulin is being absorbed through the lungs there has been some doubt about long-term safety—it would be difficult to know for many years whether inhaling insulin might impair lung function.

One preparation has been recently withdrawn from the market, but inhaled insulin may continue to be developed. Currectly there are no preparations available for use.

Insulin regimens

This is the schedule of insulin that a person will decide upon with their health-care professional, and is based on the type of diabetes, physical needs and lifestyle (in particular eating patterns and activity). The variables include type of insulin, timing, and dose. There are many regimens, but the most common examples are:

- Insulin added to oral medication. This combination is worthwhile in those with type 2 diabetes whose fasting blood glucose begins to rise despite maximum oral medication. It most often means a dose of long-acting insulin at bedtime.

- Twice daily insulin. This is either two doses of an intermediate-acting insulin or two doses of a mixed insulin to give more control over post-meal increases in blood glucose. The latter is often used in type 1 diabetes when the individual wants to avoid taking insulin at work at lunchtime.

- Basal–bolus insulin. This is essentially intensive insulin therapy and is discussed below.

Basal–bolus regimen

This is recommended for people with type 1 diabetes and some people with type 2 diabetes. It requires frequent blood glucose measurement at least before meals and at bedtime. The insulin regime usually consists of a long-acting insulin at bedtime and a dose of rapid-acting insulin before meals. The dose of the pre-meal insulin is adjusted depending on the expected carbohydrate intake which can be calculated using carbohydrate counting (see Diet in Chapter 2).

❓ FAQ

I cannot always get hold of my diabetes nurse or doctor—can I change my insulin dose myself?

Yes, but it does vary from person to person in that everyone has varying sensitivity to insulin. Here are a few tips:

- It is best to look for trends and not to treat one-off highs and lows in blood sugar. Allow 3–4 days to observe a trend.

- The basic insulin regimen should be increased by no more than 10–20% at a time and not more frequently than every 3 or 4 days.

- If recurrent hypoglycaemia occurs at the higher dose, it should be dropped back to the previous dose.

- If there is a significant change in diet and weight this can increase or decrease insulin requirements significantly.

- If no change in results is observed check your insulin, i.e. expiry and pen device, and review your injection site and technique with a healthcare professional.

Adverse effects of insulin therapy

Although insulin is no doubt life-saving to many and provides a dramatic improvement in symptoms, to others it is good to be aware of the following adverse effects:

- Hypoglycaemia. This is the most common disadvantage of insulin therapy and happens when the amount of insulin taken is too much for the amount of food ingested, exercise undertaken or starting level of blood sugar (see Chapter 4).

- Weight gain. When insulin is started, a person will begin to retain fat, which is normal to some extent; people will find they are unable to eat as much as they did previously without putting on weight and therefore they should beware of overeating. Also eating snacks to avoid hypoglycaemia should be limited as much as possible. It is usually better to reduce the insulin dose rather than eating to justify it.

- Insulin allergy. This is now extremely rare due to using human insulin.

Some special situations . . .

1. Travel

   Adjustment will be necessary when travelling through time zones that cause time changes of above 3 hours. The length of day and duration of insulin should be examined: if it is a significantly shorter day, the long-acting insulin should be omitted or reduced, and meals only covered with short-acting insulin. If the day is longer, the long-acting insulin will probably need to be supplemented with an extra short-acting injection if there are any extra meals. See Travel in Chapter 5.

2. Surgery

   People who have previously been well controlled on diet or diet and tablets may need insulin to control the blood glucose during periods of stress such as surgery.

3. Pregnancy

   This is discussed in more detail in Chapter 5. Essentially, oral medications should not be used when a woman is trying to become pregnant or is pregnant. If a woman has type 1 diabetes she will obviously continue with insulin, with it being even more crucial that there is good control for the well-being of the foetus. Insulin use is usually temporary in gestational diabetes, with the need for insulin stopping after delivery.

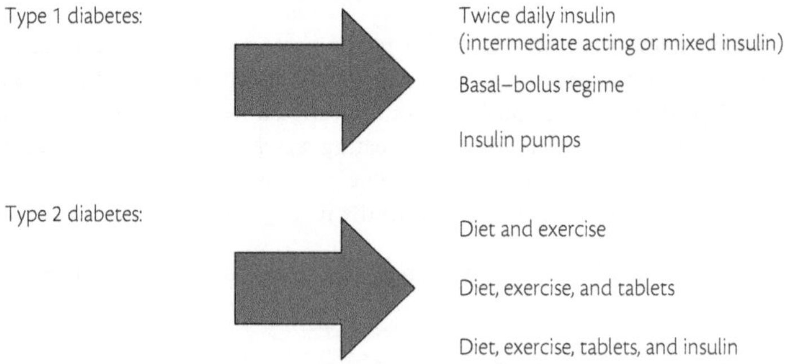

Type 1 diabetes:

Twice daily insulin
(intermediate acting or mixed insulin)

Basal–bolus regime

Insulin pumps

Type 2 diabetes:

Diet and exercise

Diet, exercise, and tablets

Diet, exercise, tablets, and insulin

Figure 3.4 Possible treatment pathways in diabetes.

4

Blood glucose levels

Monitoring glucose levels

> ### ➲ Key points
>
> ◆ Monitoring glucose levels is a useful tool for managing diabetes.
>
> ◆ Glucose levels can be monitored by testing either blood or urine.
>
> ◆ The type, timing, and frequency of blood tests will depend on the type of diabetes, treatment and an individual's lifestyle.
>
> ◆ Alternative site testing can be less painful than fingertip testing, but may not be suitable for everyone.

The monitoring of glucose levels is useful in the management of diabetes as it helps investigate the effects of medication, food, stress, illness, and physical activity on blood glucose levels. Evidence shows that maintaining blood glucose levels within target ranges may reduce the risk of the long-term complications of diabetes.

There are several methods of monitoring available which may be carried out either by the person with diabetes or by a health professional.

Glucose levels can be monitored in two main ways:

◆ By testing blood glucose levels, or

◆ By testing glucose levels in the urine.

Testing blood glucose levels

There are two principle ways of testing blood glucose levels

- **Self-monitoring of blood glucose (SMBG)**. This is a test carried out by the person with diabetes which involves pricking the side of a finger with a device to obtain a drop of blood which is then dropped onto a testing strip loaded into a hand-held blood glucose meter. There are various reliable and easy to use blood-testing meters available for people with diabetes. The frequency of testing and the type of meter to use will vary from person to person dependent on their specific needs.

- **A1c.** A1c is a test carried out by a healthcare professional that measures the amount of glycosylated haemoglobin in the blood. This test measures the long-term trend in blood glucose control. Healthcare professionals use it to help assess the progress of blood glucose management in conjunction with an individual's home blood glucose monitoring results.

> But, of course, now we've got the blood meter, it's much, much easier, much quicker and more definite indication of how your blood sugar is . . .
>
> Victor   type 1 diabetes

Why measure blood glucose levels?

SMBG may help people with diabetes to gain a better understanding of their diabetes. It is useful to:

- Look at trends and patterns in day to day blood glucose levels.

- Help determine the effects that food and exercise have on blood glucose levels.

- Help the person with diabetes understand and consequently better manage their blood glucose control.

Who should self-monitor blood glucose?

SMBG has been shown to be effective mainly for those who use insulin to treat either type 1 or type 2 diabetes, but is often used by those utilizing other methods to treat their diabetes. It may be useful to discuss the most appropriate method of monitoring blood glucose with a healthcare professional. The areas that may be discussed are:

- Whether there is a clinical need for self-monitoring.

- How frequently blood glucose levels should be tested.

- How the results are going to be used.

The clinical need for self-monitoring

Evidence has shown that the people in the following groups show most benefit from regular SMBG:

- All people with type 1 diabetes.

- Women with type 1 or 2 diabetes who are pregnant or planning pregnancy.

- Women with gestational diabetes.

- Type 2 diabetes treated by combined insulin and oral hypoglycaemic agents.

There is currently some debate about the effectiveness of regular blood glucose monitoring in those whose diabetes is treated by any other oral hypoglycaemic medication or diet and lifestyle, and the current consensus for this group is that if stable, regular measurement of A1c is a suitable way of monitoring blood glucose levels. This recommendation may change if blood glucose levels are unstable or if diabetes treatment is changed.

> ## ❓ FAQ
>
> **I have been diagnosed with type 2 diabetes but I don't take any tablets to treat it. Should I measure my blood glucose every day?**
>
> No, regular tests of your A1c level should be enough to monitor your blood glucose levels. However, if your symptoms change, or you start to take tablets or insulin to treat your diabetes, this may change.

How frequently should blood glucose levels be tested?

Frequency of SMBG will depend on the way diabetes is treated and will be affected by lifestyle and the requirements of the person with diabetes. The following table gives some general guidelines, but it will be important to discuss the frequency of testing and any resulting actions with a healthcare professional.

Treatment regimen	Frequency of testing
Twice daily insulin	Twice daily at various times in order to identify any trends
Basal–bolus	4 times a day
Insulin pump therapy	4–6 times a day
Pregnant or planning pregnancy, gestational diabetes	4–6 times a day, although this may need to be more intensive dependent on circumstances
Combined insulin and oral hypoglycaemic therapy	At least once daily. It is recommended that tests are done at various times on each day to help identify any patterns in blood glucose levels
Sulphonylureas alone or with other anti-diabetic medication	Frequency of testing will vary dependent on symptoms experienced. As a general guideline, it is recommended that testing is carried out three times a week at different times on each day
Diet and exercise	Guidelines suggest that SMBG in this group of patients would only be necessary in special circumstances, e.g. during illness or when treatment is changed

How useful are the results?

Results from SMBG can be extremely useful in identifying patterns or trends in blood glucose levels and may help the person with diabetes achieve a better understanding and consequently provide a tool to help them manage their diabetes. To help identify any patterns, it is useful to record the results in either a paper- or computer-based diary and to ensure that testing, especially if done only a few times a week, is done at different times each day.

Which blood glucose meter to use

There are many types of meter on the market, ranging from very simple to very complex. Most meters are available to buy in high-street pharmacies, and strips may be supplied on prescription. Determining which blood glucose meter to use is best done after discussion with a healthcare professional. For those with visual problems there are talking meters available.

	Insulin type, dose, and injection time					Blood glucose levels					Comments
Date											

Figure 4.1 An example of a self-monitoring diary.

The main points to consider when choosing a meter are:

Size: of both the meter and the visual display.

Complexity: there is wide variation in how much information the meter will provide. This ranges from a simple readout and number memory to the facility to work with a computer and to draw graphs to help establish trends.

Amount of blood: although most meters require a very small amount of blood to test, some require more than others.

Alternative site testing: some meters come with a device that will allow testing of sites other than the fingertip.

Safety: some meters come with pre-loaded lancet and strips allowing for safe disposal of used strips and needles.

How to test blood glucose levels using a hand-held meter

The minimum requirements for SMBG are:

- A suitable meter that the person with diabetes feels comfortable using.

- Testing strips that work with the meter.

- A lancet (finger-pricking) device to obtain blood from the fingertip or other testing area.

- Facilities where hands can be washed before testing.

After carefully washing and drying hands, a finger prick device is held against the side of the selected finger. The drop of blood is then applied to a testing strip and, after a short period of time, the meter will display the blood glucose level. The results on the meter are expressed in millimoles per litre (mmol/l).

Top tips for blood glucose testing

Wash hands   Wash hands first and dry well—dirt, food, and liquids can affect meter readings.

Warm hands   Improve blood flow by running hands under warm water and massaging the finger before testing.

Test on the side   Select a site on the side of the finger rather than the tip. The sides are less sensitive.

Change lancet regularly   Use a new lancet every time—reusing lancets can make testing painful.

Change sites   Use different fingers each time—this allows fingers to recover between tests.

Set lancing device to correct setting   Skin thickness can affect how deeply the lancet should pierce the skin—choosing a lance that has various depth settings can minimize pain that may be felt when testing.

What do the results mean?

Diabetes UK currently recommends that people with diabetes aim to keep their blood levels at:

- 4–6 mmol/l before meals (preprandial).

- No higher than 10 mmol/l at 2 hours after meals (postprandial).

Evidence shows that staying within these targets can help to reduce the risk of long-term complications associated with diabetes.

Disposal of sharps

It is important that any sharp lancing device that is used to obtain the blood sample from the finger or alternative site is disposed of safely. It is important that the sharps are collected in a special 'sharps' box. People with diabetes should ask a member of their healthcare team for advice on the most appropriate methods of storage and disposal of lancets and needles for their area.

Alternative site testing

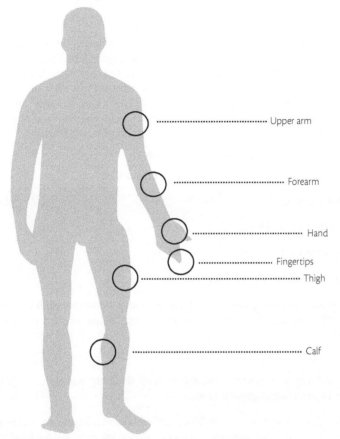

··· Upper arm

··· Forearm

··· Hand

···························· Fingertips

······························· Thigh

··· Calf

Figure 4.2 Alternative sites for blood glucose testing.

Some meters are supplied with a lancet device that will allow blood to be obtained from sites other than the fingertip. Sometimes people feel that frequent testing on the fingertips is painful or may result in calloused fingertips. Other body sites such as the forearm have fewer pain receptors than the fingertips.

When alternative site testing is recommended

At times when blood glucose levels are stable, for example:

◆ Immediately before a meal.

◆ When fasting.

◆ Near bedtime.

It is important to note that when blood glucose levels are changing rapidly, there may be a difference in the glucose readings between the finger and other test sites, e.g. the forearm, upper arm, thigh, calf, and other areas of the hand. Because blood flow to the finger is 3–5 times faster than to other sites, blood samples from the finger may show changes in blood glucose sooner than an alternative testing site. The possible difference in glucose readings between the finger and other sites could delay the detection of hypoglycaemia.

When alternative site testing is not recommended

◆ After food when blood glucose is rising quickly.

◆ After exercise.

◆ During times of illness.

◆ To detect hypoglyceamia.

◆ Hypoglycaemia unawareness (see page 93).

Alternative site testing should be discussed with a healthcare professional to establish the suitability of this method of blood testing for the person with diabetes.

A1c

A1c, or haemoglobin A1c, is the abbreviation for a test that measures glycosylated haemoglobin levels in blood.

Haemoglobin is a protein of the blood cells that carries oxygen to cells in the body. As glucose circulates in the bloodstream it sticks to the haemoglobin molecule, converting it into glycosylated haemoglobin. When glucose levels in blood become raised, more glucose sticks to the haemoglobin molecule, raising the glycosylated haemoglobin or A1c level. As the life of a haemoglobin molecule is about 2–3 months, it gives a good idea of the average quantity of glucose in the blood over the same period. This can help determine how well a person's diabetes is being controlled in that time.

As this test relies on normal levels of haemoglobin, for those with conditions such as anaemia, thalassaemia or sickle cell anaemia (conditions which involve a lack of or abnormal type of haemoglobin), the A1c may not be a true reflection of long-term glucose levels. Other tests are available for people with these conditions, and this should be discussed with a healthcare professional.

How A1c is tested

This test is carried out by a health professional. Blood is drawn from a vein in the arm or hand, and then sent to a laboratory for analysis.

What do the results mean?

The results of the test are expressed as a percentage. The aim of diabetes treatment is to lower the A1c to below a target level, and current evidence shows that if the level of A1c is below 6.5% then the risk of complications such as eye disease, kidney disease, heart disease, and nerve damage are reduced.

However, if there are problems with severe hypoglycaemia, then a target level of 7.5% is recommended.

❓ FAQ

My doctor says I need an A1c test every 6 months, but I don't take any medication to treat my diabetes—why do I need this done?

This test shows the approximate level of blood glucose over the past 2–3 months. By doing the test, the doctor can tell if blood glucose levels are changing and if treatment needs to be changed to keep blood glucose levels in the normal range

I test my blood glucose level four times a day—why do I need an A1c test as well?

The A1c test will give the health professional a picture of overall glucose control. The tests that are done at home only give a picture of what blood glucose is at any one time, whereas the A1c gives a picture of your average blood glucose control for the past 2–3 months. The results give you a good idea of how well your diabetes treatment plan is working.

Testing glucose levels in the urine

When the level of glucose in blood rises above normal levels, the kidneys eliminate the excess glucose in the urine. Glucose in urine, therefore, reflects an excess of glucose in blood.

A urine glucose test involves holding a test strip in the stream of urine for a few seconds and, after a defined time, comparing the colour on the strip with the chart provided. Each colour represents a certain blood glucose level.

When to test urine

The optimal time to test levels of glucose in the urine is in the morning before breakfast. It is best to empty the bladder first and then test a sample passed about 30 minutes later. A urine test carried out first thing will only give levels of glucose in the urine that has been stored in the bladder overnight and will not give an accurate reflection of recent glucose levels.

> ### ❓ FAQ
>
> ## So is it better to test urine or blood glucose levels?
>
> Monitoring glucose levels can be achieved by blood or urine testing. The advantages and disadvantages of each method are outlined in the table below

Type	Advantages	Disadvantages
Urine testing	Simple to use No need to prick finger to obtain sample Inexpensive	Less accurate than testing blood as there is normally no glucose in the urine until the blood glucose level has risen to more than 10 mmol/l Unsuitable for those on insulin or sulphonyureas as low blood glucose levels cannot be detected Cannot determine accurate times of blood glucose levels May be impractical due to travelling, work, etc.
Blood glucose monitoring (SMBG)	Effective, simple and convenient method Practical to use in different situations, e.g. work or travelling Provides 'real-time' results which may help when: ◆ making food choices ◆ making choices about driving or exercise Recording blood glucose level results will help identify patterns that may inform changes in medication and identify hypo- and hyperglycaemia	More expensive than urine testing May be painful May not be clinically effective if not treated by insulin

(continued)

Type	Advantages	Disadvantages
A1c (glycated haemoglobin)	A good way of monitoring longer term control of blood glucose levels Less frequent testing; testing is recommended every 2–6 months for people with type 2 diabetes.	Involves a visit to a healthcare professional for a blood sample to be taken Not suitable as the only testing method for those using insulin to treat diabetes; regular blood glucose monitoring using a meter is recommended for this group of patients If there are extremes in day-to-day blood glucose levels this will not be reflected in the A1c result

➜ Summary

Testing glucose levels can be useful for people with diabetes, although the evidence is limited. People with diabetes require an understanding of their glucose levels, and this involves patient education. A close working relationship between the person with diabetes and their health professional can support decision making around the management and control of glucose levels.

Hypoglycaemia

➜ Key points

- There are various causes, signs, and symptoms of hypoglycaemia

- Hypoglycaemia should be treated as soon as possible

- Hypoglycaemic unawareness can increase the risk of a hypo and can affect health and quality of life

What is hypoglycaemia?

Hypoglycaemia is generally accepted to be a blood glucose level below 4 mmol/l and is often referred to as a 'hypo'. People who take insulin and/or certain tablets called sulphonylureas are at risk of having a hypo, but hypos are less common for those on tablets than for those on insulin. Those people who are treated with just diet alone or a tablet known as metformin do not develop any significant hypoglycaemia.

It is essential that those with diabetes understand the signs, symptoms and causes of hypos, and that their family are aware of what to do in the event of a hypo. When a hypo happens it can be an alarming experience, but not necessarily life threatening.

Causes of hypoglycaemia

- Taking too much diabetes medication, either insulin or certain tablets.

- Missing or delaying a meal or snack.

- Eating less carbohydrate than normal.

- More activity or exercise than normal.

- Drinking alcohol without carbohydrate.

❓ FAQ

When I am on holiday and sunbathing on the beach, I often have a hypo. How is this possible? I am not exercising, which I know can often lower my blood glucose levels.

When lying in the sun, the insulin you have previously injected is absorbed at a faster rate. This is due to the small blood vessels under the skin dilating in response to heat. Either a reduction in your insulin dose or taking extra carbohydrate will help reduce the risk of a hypo while sun bathing.

Signs and symptoms

. . . So long as there are early warning signs of a hypo, and I can take a couple of glucose tablets, that's fine, there's no problem, and I need involve nobody.

Phillip, type 1 diabetes   www.diabetes-stories.com

As the glucose levels fall, there are 'warning signs' that occur as the body tries to raise the blood glucose levels. These warning signs can vary from person to person, and have two separate effects. The first are symptoms caused by the release of adrenaline in response to low blood glucose (adrenergic response) and the second is a lack of blood glucose to the brain (neuroglycopenia). Signs and symptoms can be classified as mild, moderate, or severe.

Symptoms of mild hypoglycaemia

This is the body's first-line response to falling blood glucose levels. As blood glucose levels fall, the hormone adrenaline is released from the adrenal glands above the kidney, and this causes the liver to release stored glucose into the bloodstream. Adrenaline also causes the 'fight or flight' response, creating some of the same symptoms that occur during frightening situations. These symptoms are:

- Sweating

- Trembling

- Palpitations

- Anxiety

- Blurred vision

- Hunger

- Tiredness

- Headache

Symptoms of moderate hypoglycaemia

If the hypo continues untreated, the brain becomes affected by a lack of glucose and begins to shut down. This can be a frightening experience, as these symptoms can lead to a feeling of loss of control. Of course, it is less likely that a person with diabetes will be able to treat him or herself at this point and they may need help from others. The symptoms of moderate hypos are:

- Lack of co-ordination

- Speech difficulty

- Drowsiness

- Confusion

- Aggression

Symptoms of severe hypoglycaemia

> . . . if I go hypo, seriously hypo, or I don't know that I've gone, it tends to be in the early hours of the morning—and a couple of years ago—I must have been groaning—my ten-year-old daughter actually came in and she saw me going hypo and got actually quite scared about it.
>
> Mary, type 1 diabetes   www.diabetes-stories.com

Hypoglycaemia that remains untreated causes the brain to shut down and can result in:

- Convulsions

- Coma

Severe hypoglycaemia will need medical treatment as the swallowing reflex is not operating and so treatment using food and drink is impossible. Partners or relatives may be able to help treat people who are unconscious.

Advice for treating severe hypoglycaemia

If an individual is unconscious, place them in the recovery position to keep their airway clear. Do not attempt to put glucose or fluid into the mouth of someone who is unconscious. If the person is unable to swallow, a friend or relative can give a glucagon injection. Glucagon is a hormone that raises blood glucose levels by releasing glucose stores from the liver. Glucagon needs to be dissolved in a solvent in a pre-filled syringe given deep into muscle (e.g. the thigh). This can also be given as an injection into a vein or under the skin. It is available on prescription and it may be reassuring to keep some at home for friends or relatives to give in severe circumstances. Glucagon has only a short-acting effect, so the individual will need some sugar by mouth on waking, to maintain a normal blood glucose level. If they do not respond to glucagon, then intravenous glucose is required. It will usually be necessary to call an ambulance or doctor.

If a glucagon injection is not available, or there are problems administering it, call an ambulance immediately.

Treating hypoglycaemia

Mild or moderate hypoglycaemia

- Treat symptoms as soon as possible.

- Test blood glucose levels if circumstances allow.

- If this is not possible, treat the conditions as for a hypo.

- In general, 15 g of fast-acting carbohydrate, followed by 15 g of slower-acting carbohydrate are adequate.

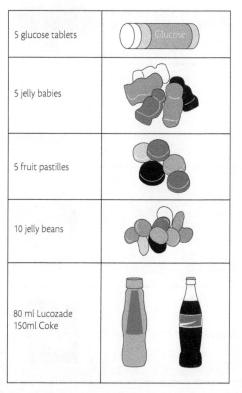

5 glucose tablets	
5 jelly babies	
5 fruit pastilles	
10 jelly beans	
80 ml Lucozade 150ml Coke	

Figure 4.3 Treatment for hypoglyaemia. These foods and drinks supply 15 g of fast-acting carbohydrate.

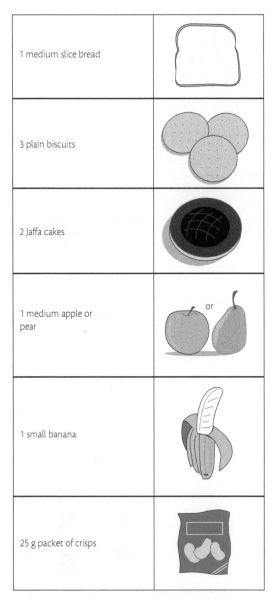

1 medium slice bread	
3 plain biscuits	
2 Jaffa cakes	
1 medium apple or pear	
1 small banana	
25 g packet of crisps	

Figure 4.4 Treatment for hypoglycaemia. These foods and drinks supply 15 g of slower-acting carbohydrate.

The rule of 15 is a useful way to remember the most efficient way to treat a hypo.

The rule of 15

Step 1

Take 15 g of fast-acting glucose (e.g. jelly beans, glucose, Lucozade)

Step 2

If the next meal is not due within the next 15–20 minutes, follow step 1 by 15 g of longer-acting carbohydrate (e.g. biscuits, sandwich)

Step 3

Wait 10–15 minutes. If the blood glucose levels do not rise to normal levels, repeat step 1.

IT IS IMPORTANT TO TREAT A HYPO IMMEDIATELY TO STOP FURTHER REDUCTIONS IN BLOOD GLUCOSE LEVELS

Treatment for preventing hypos

◆ Avoid skipping meals.

◆ Record any episodes of hypoglycaemia in your blood glucose diary and investigate possible reasons for hypoglycaemia.

◆ Try to identify the cause of the hypo in order to prevent it happening again.

◆ If hypos are occurring frequently, contact a doctor or diabetes nurse.

◆ Always carry fast-acting glucose with you.

◆ It is advisable to test blood glucose levels before driving (the levels should be above 4 mmol/l before driving).

◆ Eat carbohydrate if you are drinking alcohol on an empty stomach.

Hypoglycaemia unawareness

. . . I don't seem to get the symptoms that people are supposed to experience, and when you do, you have a few minutes in which to react, otherwise it's too late.

Phillip   type 1 diabetes

Hypoglycaemic unawareness is a condition in which people no longer experience the usual warning signs of hypoglycaemia. The symptoms of hypoglycaemia may be different, less pronounced or even absent. Hypo unawareness is more prevalent in people with type 1 diabetes.

The effects of hypoglycaemia unawareness

There are real dangers concerning hypoglycaemic unawareness. It can affect relationships and family life, work, and ability to drive. There is mounting evidence to support the theory that repeated moderate/severe hypos can lead to reduced cognitive function. Hypoglycaemia unawareness is a situation best managed in conjunction with a doctor or diabetes nurse specialist.

It is essential for those who have hypo unawareness to inform the DVLA and, in some circumstances, it may be advisable to stop driving (see Chapter 5).

Hypoglycaemia unawareness can result in the following:

◆ Loss of driving licence. It is illegal to drive if there is a loss of hypoglycaemic warning symptoms.

◆ Being unable to work/lack of support in employment situations.

◆ Feeling out of control.

◆ Aggressive behaviour.

◆ Detrimental effect on relationships.

What are the causes?

An increased frequency of hypoglycaemia can cause lack of awareness. This includes hypos occurring at night, when symptoms may not be recognized and are slept through. In those people who have frequent hypoglycaemia it may be that the brain resets itself to recognize lower levels of blood glucose as hypoglycaemia.

A long duration of diabetes can cause hypoglycaemia unawareness. People who have 'tight' blood glucose levels, meaning blood glucose levels that are frequently in the normal to low range, are also at risk.

Many people feel strongly that converting from animal insulin (especially pork insulin) to human insulin has contributed to the loss of warning symptoms. There is little evidence that this is the case, although much research has taken place in this area. If people with diabetes feel strongly that the change from animal to human insulin has reduced their warning symptoms, alternative forms of insulin are available. These include either the pork version of the insulin currently taken, or perhaps one of the new insulin analogues (see Chapter 3). People often report that hypo symptoms return after a change to animal insulin.

If looking at the blood glucose diary indicates no obvious reason for the loss of awareness, then night-time hypos, which can go unrecognized while asleep, may be the cause. Hypoglycaemia occurring during the night is of great concern for people with diabetes who are insulin treated, but even if a hypo occurs and is not recognized, the blood glucose will normally rise again overnight as the body runs out of insulin.

? FAQ

I have read about hypos happening during sleep. What would happen if I had a hypo while asleep—would I wake up?

The reaction to a hypo during sleep depends on the individual. Some people find that a hypo wakes them. They may have vivid dreams or wake sweaty and confused. Other people sleep straight through a hypo and wake feeling 'hungover', or with a headache. Routine checking of blood sugar levels at 3.00 a.m. may detect unsuspected night-time hypos.

How can lost hypo warnings be restored?

This need not be a permanent state. It may be advisable to maintain higher glucose levels in the short term, for at least a month, and this may encourage the return to an awareness of hypo symptoms.

How to reduce the risk of hypo unawareness

- Maintain blood glucose levels at a higher level. This usually means reducing the insulin dose.

- Do blood glucose tests regularly.

- Always test before driving.

- Ensure friends and family know what a hypo is and what action to take. Consider having a glucagon kit available.

Those people who have hypo unawareness may consider informing others that they have diabetes, especially family and friends. This situation also highlights the need for ID tags or bracelets (available from Diabetes UK) so that others can identify an individual with diabetes.

Hyperglycaemia

➜ Key points

- Hyperglycaemia is usually associated with illness and infections.

- Ketoacidosis can occur in people with type 1 diabetes and is usually associated with hyperglycaemia and illness.

- Diabetic ketoacidosis is potentially a serious condition which needs immediate action.

- It is important to drink plenty of clear fluids if hyperglycaemia or ketoacidosis are present, and to maintain usual carbohydrate intake with either food or drink if possible.

- Medication, especially insulin, should not be stopped or reduced in illness.

What is hyperglycaemia?

Hyperglycaemia means a high blood glucose level. Blood glucose levels in the range 4–8 mmol/l are generally accepted to be normal. A reading of 10 mmol/l and above is considered a hyperglycaemic level.

What is ketoacidosis?

Ketoacidosis occurs in those with type 1 diabetes and is related to the production of substances called ketones. When there is not enough insulin in the body, glucose cannot be used by the cells to provide enough energy. The body then resorts to burning fat to obtain this energy, and the process causes ketones to be produced. Ketones can be used as energy by the body, and the brain can use them in starvation when there is no glucose available. However, the build up of moderate or large amounts of ketones in the urine and blood is dangerous and disturbs the chemical balance in the blood. Eventually, the rise in ketone levels causes the blood to become acidic, which is known as diabetic ketoacidosis (DKA).

What causes high blood glucose levels?

The most common causes of high blood glucose levels are:

- Illness

- Infection

- Stress

- Large amounts of carbohydrate with insufficient medication

- Side effects relating to some medications, e.g. steroids

Sometimes there may be no identifiable cause for raised blood glucose levels. However, in response to illness, the body produces a stress hormone called 'cortisol' that causes blood glucose levels to rise. Common illnesses that can increase blood glucose levels are: sore throats, gastroenteritis, diarrhoea, and urine infections.

Symptoms of hyperglycaemia

> . . . for me personally high blood sugars has always meant extreme thirst, very dry mouth, dizziness and feeling sick. There has always been a distinct difference between that feeling and low blood sugar levels.
>
> Joanne, type 1 diabetes   www.diabetes-stories.com

Initial symptoms	Later symptoms
Thirst	Nausea/vomiting
Dry mouth	Loss of appetite and weakness
Passing more urine	Dehydration
High blood glucose readings	Confusion
	Blurred vision
	People with type 1 diabetes may go on to develop ketoacidosis with these symptoms:
	Fruity odour on the breath
	Abdominal pain
	Rapid breathing
	Weight loss

Symptoms of hyperglycaemia are similar to those of untreated diabetes. The symptoms can appear either slowly over a period of days, or suddenly over a few hours. People with diabetes who feel unwell are advised to test blood glucose levels regularly as this will give an indication if hyperglycaemia is occurring.

Treatment of high blood glucose levels

Type 1 diabetes: sick-day rules

As people with type 1 diabetes are at risk of developing DKA, it is important to take action at the earliest possible sign of any form of illness such as a cold, infection or a virus. Regular monitoring of blood glucose levels is advised and insulin doses may need to be increased if necessary. Those with type 1 diabetes are also advised to check for the presence of ketones.

How can I test for ketones?

It is possible to check for ketones in the urine or blood. The ketones build up in the bloodstream and spill over into the urine causing 'ketonuria' which can be detected by dipping a test strip in the urine and reading the colour. The test strips are available on prescription.

Many people with type 1 diabetes can benefit from measuring blood ketones using a special meter, which can detect levels of ketones in the blood. It is advisable to contact a diabetes nurse or doctor for further advice on this method of testing for ketones. Again, the strips are available on prescription.

People with type 1 diabetes should test their urine or blood for ketones if their blood glucose levels are high (usually over 14 mmol/l) or if they are developing symptoms of ketoacidosis. DKA or ketoacidosis can develop and progress quickly. The treatment for advanced DKA may require admission to hospital. However, it is possible to prevent ketoacidosis by recognizing the warning signs, checking the urine and blood regularly for ketones and glucose, and treating with extra insulin.

What action should be taken if blood glucose levels are high?
Guidelines

Guidelines for extra insulin to treat hyperglycaemia or raised ketones depend upon the total daily dose of insulin taken by the individual. This can be calculated by adding together all the long- and short-acting insulin taken over 24 hours. The table below provides guidance for people with type 1 diabetes who are taking four or more injections a day (known as the basal–bolus or basal–prandial regimen).

Blood glucose level	Ketone level	Action
More than 14 mmol/l	0–1 mmol/l	Take extra short-acting insulin immediately: **5–10%** of total daily dose
More than 14 mmol/l	1–3 mmol/l	Take extra short-acting insulin immediately: **10–20%** of total daily dose
More than 14 mmol/l	More than 3 mmol/l	Take extra short-acting insulin: **10–20%** of total daily dose and seek medical help immediately

If ketones are present, monitoring and treatment should be repeated at hourly intervals until blood glucose and ketone levels begin to come down.

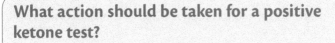

What action should be taken for a positive ketone test?

- Take extra rapid-acting insulin as soon as possible (see table above).

- Drink plenty of water and unsweetened fluids.

- Test blood glucose every 1–2 hours and repeat the extra insulin (see table above) until blood/urine is negative to ketones.

- Try to identify cause of high blood glucose level and seek treatment if necessary.

- Contact diabetes team if high glucose and ketone levels persist.

- Contact GP/Accident and Emergency Department if you are vomiting, as dehydration may occur.

- Continue with the usual amount of background insulin.

REMEMBER—drink at least a cupful of unsweetened fluid every 15 minutes (about 500 ml per hour) while blood glucose levels are high

ALWAYS—take insulin during times of illness

❓ FAQ

What action should be taken for high blood glucose leels with a negative ketone test?

- Continue to test for ketones every 1–2 hours while blood glucose levels remain above 14 mmol/l.

- If ketone test becomes positive treat as above.

- If ketone test is negative, but blood glucose levels remain above 14 mmol/l, treat with insulin (see table above).

- Drink plenty of water and unsweetened fluids.

- Try to identify the cause of high blood glucose level and seek treatment if necessary.

- Continue with the usual amount of background insulin.

❓ FAQ

Can I reduce my blood glucose levels by doing more exercise?

Blood glucose levels can be reduced by exercise when ketones are absent. However, the presence of ketones in someone with type 1 diabetes shows a dangerous lack of insulin, which should be corrected immediately. Exercise at this time will only burn more fat and produce more ketones. If hyperglycaemia or ketones are caused by illness or infection, it is advisable not to exercise.

Doing the maths for my insulin alteration when I am ill seems really complicated. Is there a way to make the maths easier?

Some people find it easy to do the calculations when they are feeling well, but difficult when they are unwell. If this is the case for you, then it may be worth making a note of the figures for 5%, 10%, and 20% of your total daily insulin dose for future reference.

Type 2 diabetes

People with type 2 diabetes tend to experience the initial symptoms of hyperglycaemia (see symptoms table), but will not develop ketoacidosis.

It is normal for blood glucose levels to go up and down from day to day. An occasional high blood glucose level is not a problem. Blood glucose levels may remain high for a longer period of time in the presence of illness or infection. Illness causes the body to become more resistant to insulin and increases the amount of insulin required, especially during periods of illness. In addition, a stress hormone, 'cortisol', will cause the blood glucose levels to rise. People with type 2 diabetes treated by tablets do not usually have the option to increase their dose over the short-term to lower blood glucose levels and are advised to contact their healthcare team for advice. People treated by insulin may need more insulin during periods of illness and should contact their healthcare team for advice and support. Generally, it is considered safe to change a dose by 10%.

For individuals who are not ill, but who have consistently high blood glucose levels, two possible changes in medication are common. Either their medication can be increased in order to reduce blood glucose levels, or they may need to commence insulin if they are already on the optimum dose of their diabetes tablets.

Type 2 diabetes: sick-day rules

What action to take when unwell

- Test blood glucose levels at least every 2–4 hours.

- Keep drinking and take some carbohydrate as either food or drink if possible. This action will avoid hypoglycaemia and prevent dehydration. If eating normally, sip unsweetened fluids, e.g. water, diet soft drinks, and tea. If unable to eat normally, drink sweetened fluids, e.g. fruit juice, milk, and tea or coffee with added sugar.

- Do not stop taking any diabetes medication.

- If the person with diabetes is not able to manage their diabetes during times of illness, it is essential to ask for help and call a doctor or diabetes nurse.

> REMEMBER—it is important to keep up fluid levels and carbohydrates when ill. Never stop diabetes medication.

When to call a doctor

- If unable to eat normally and requiring advice on diabetes medication doses.

- If an individual is not well enough to follow 'sick-day rules'.

- If blood glucose levels are consistently above 15 mmol/l for more than 12 hours.

- If vomiting or diarrhoea continue for more than 12 hours.

- If the person with diabetes becomes drowsy or increasingly unwell.

Those with type 2 diabetes who experience very high blood glucose levels—often over 40 mmol/l—can develop a condition called hyperosmolar non-ketotic acidosis (HONK).

5

Living with diabetes

Driving

People with either type 1 or type 2 diabetes are usually able to continue driving, but the following factors need consideration:

◆ The law about driving and diabetes.

◆ Driving and restricted licences.

◆ Driving and insurance.

◆ Safety aspects, including hypoglycaemia and problems with eyesight.

The law regarding driving and diabetes

People with diabetes who are treated by diet and/or oral hypoglycaemic tablets can continue to drive with their normal licence until they are 70. This is usually referred to as keeping their 'until 70' licence. However, the Driver and Vehicle Licensing Agency (DVLA) must, by law, be informed when:

◆ Treatment with insulin is required.

◆ The person with diabetes is treated by insulin and applying for a licence for the first time.

◆ Any laser treatment to the eyes for retinopathy is required.

◆ Any eye is affected by other eye problems (excluding short/long sight or colour blindness). The law requires that the driver must be able to read, with corrective lenses if necessary, a car number plate in good light at 20.5 metres (67 feet) or 20 metres (65 feet) where narrower characters 50 mm wide are displayed.

◆ Problems develop with the circulation or sensation in the legs, which make it necessary to drive certain types of vehicles only, e.g. automatic vehicles or those with modifications such as a hand-operated accelerator/brake. This must be noted on the licence.

◆ Any existing medical condition deteriorates or any condition develops that may affect safe driving at any time in the future. This includes the complications of diabetes; frequent hypoglycaemic episodes that are likely to impair driving, loss or impaired hypoglycaemic awareness, eyesight complications that affect visual acuity or visual fields, and limb disability including peripheral neuropathy.

The DVLA recommends that if diabetes is treated by tablets then they should be informed, even if no relevant complications exist. This allows the DVLA to keep the person with diabetes fully informed of future requirements.

In Northern Ireland, the rules differ slightly in that people diagnosed with diabetes and treated with oral hypoglycaemic tablets must inform the Driver and Vehicle Agency (DVA). For other countries, the appropriate government licensing body should be contacted for the specific laws regarding diabetes and driving.

❓ FAQ

What happens if I already have a driving licence?

If any of the above criteria are fulfilled, then you must inform the DVLA immediately and not wait until your driving licence is due for renewal.

What happens if I apply for a new licence?

You will be asked health questions as part of the normal application and you will be asked to give details about your treatment. After the licence application has been completed and returned, another form (DIAB1) will be sent asking for more detailed information and the name of your GP or diabetes specialist. This will include a consent form which will allow the DVLA to approach your healthcare professional directly so that a medical report can be obtained.

Decisions that may be made

Once all the medical information has been made available, a decision will be made about the issue of a driving licence. The following are the possible outcomes:

◆ The licence will be retained or a new licence will be issued.

◆ A driving licence will be issued for a period of 1, 2 or 3 years if a medical advisor decides that a review of medical fitness is required.

◆ A driving licence may be issued that requires special controls be fitted to the vehicle being driven.

◆ The driving licence may be revoked or refused. This will only happen if the enquiries made confirm that the medical standards of fitness to drive are not met as a result of a medical condition. If this happens, the person will be provided with a reason for the decision, informed when they may re-apply and sent notice of their right to appeal.

These procedures do not mean a diagnosis of diabetes leads to refusal or loss of a driving licence. The DVLA ensures that every licensed driver is safe to drive and if someone is living with diabetes that is well controlled, and where there are no complications that might impair safe driving, there is no reason why a licence should not be issued.

Driving and restricted licences

Current legislation is such that if insulin is used for the treatment of diabetes, it is against the law to have or hold a LGV (Large Goods Vehicle) or PCV (Passenger Carrying Vehicle) licence. There are two licence groups:

Group 1: this includes car and motorcycles.

Group 2: this includes large lorries and buses. The medical standards in this group are higher because of the size and weight of the vehicle. They reflect the increased risk caused by the length of time the driver spends at the wheel as a result of their occupation.

Tables 5.1 and 5.2 outline the requirements for licence issue for each group of drivers, based on treatment and presence of complications.

Table 5.1 Licence entitlements based on diabetes complications

Diabetes complications	Group 1 Cars and motorcyles	Group 2 Lorries and buses
Frequent hypoglycaemic episodes that are likely to affect driving	Must stop driving until satisfactory control is maintained. This will be subject to a medical report.	**If a** licence holder, must stop driving until satisfactory control is maintained. This will be subject to a medical report.
Hypoglycaemic unawareness	Driving must stop if this is confirmed. Driving may be resumed if hypoglycaemic awareness regained and this is confirmed by a medical report.	**If a** licence holder, must stop driving. Driving may be resumed if hypoglycaemic awareness regained and this is confirmed by a medical report.
Eyesight complications	Must be able to meet the legal eyesight requirements.	Must be able to meet the legal eyesight requirements.
Limb disability e.g. peripheral neuropathy	Driving is possible, and the DVLA must be informed of these complications. Vehicle modification may be necessary.	Some disabilities **may** be compatible with the driving of large vehicles if mild and non-progressive. Individual assessment will be required.

Table 5.2 Licence entitlements based on diabetes treatment

Diabetes treatment	Group 1 Cars and motorcyles	Group 2 Lorries and buses
Insulin	Must recognize warning symptoms of hypoglycaemia.	New applicants or existing drivers on insulin must not drive HGV or PCV vehicles. Drivers with licences issued before 1 April 1991 are dealt with on an individual basis and are subject to annual review. Changes in regulations mean that since 2001, 'exceptional case' drivers are allowed to apply or renew their entitlement to drive small lorries subject to meeting qualifying conditions.
Oral hypoglycaemic tablets	May continue to hold 'until 70' licence unless relevant complications develop.	Drivers may retain their licence unless complications lead to relevant disabilities such as problems with eyes that would mean the legal requirements for eyesight are not met. If treatment changes and insulin is required, the rules or insulin treatment apply.
Diet alone	No notification needed unless relevant disabilities develop, e.g. eye problems Driving is possible, and the DVLA must be informed of these complications. Vehicle modification may be neccessary.	No notification needed unless relevant disabilities develop, e.g. eye problems Some disabilities may be compatible with the driving of large vehicles if mild and non-progressive. Individual assessment will be required.

❓ FAQ

New drugs to treat diabetes are coming onto the market at the moment. What happens if I am prescribed one of these?

It would be recommended that you contact the DVLA. It is important that the licensing agency and your insurers are informed of any changes in treatment.

Other driving restrictions

Driving taxis

Licences to drive a taxi have traditionally been dependent on local authority guidelines. In 2006 the Department of Transport issued new guidelines for England and Wales that recommended the application of specific standards to taxi and PCV drivers treated with insulin. This means that licences should be issued annually following strict medical assessment.

Driving emergency vehicles

Current legislation recommends that drivers who use insulin to treat diabetes should not drive emergency vehicles. The reason given for this is that it may be difficult for an individual to monitor blood glucose levels in an emergency situation.

Driving and insurance

A diagnosis of diabetes, regardless of treatment, must be disclosed either at the time of diagnosis or at the start of a new policy. At the time of renewal, any changing treatment for development of new complications must also be disclosed. Failure to notify the insurer may invalidate any claim made.

Diabetes and safe driving

> I check my blood sugars much more regularly now, because, obviously, the gadgets are available. I'm driving, so I'm much more aware of what my levels are.
>
> Lisa   type 1 diabetes

The most relevant driving hazard for drivers with diabetes is hypoglycaemia ('hypo'), especially if the person with diabetes is treated with insulin or certain diabetes tablets. It is against the law to drive if there is reduced awareness of hypoglycaemia.

Tips to avoid hypoglycaemia while driving

- Check blood glucose levels before the journey and treat if necessary.

- It is recommended that you stop every 2 hours on a long journey, check blood glucose levels and take appropriate action.

◆ Keep fast-acting glucose at hand, **not** in the glove compartment. This may be glucose tablets, Lucozade or jelly beans, and follow the '15 rule' (this is explained in full in Chapter 4).

Tips for managing hypoglycaemia while driving

◆ Stop driving as soon as it is safe to do so.

◆ Take fast-acting glucose immediately.

◆ Leave the driving seat taking the ignition key. It is important to make clear that you are not in charge of the car as a driver may be charged with driving under the influence of a drug if found in the driving seat during a hypoglycaemic episode.

◆ Wait for 15 minutes and retest blood glucose level, treat as necessary and continue until blood glucose levels return to the normal range.

If the person with diabetes has impaired or no warnings of hypoglycaemia, the law states that they should not drive. This may be reassessed, and the DVLA will only issue a licence if a supporting medical report is provided.

> Some statistics:
> Crashes among type 1 diabetic drivers were associated with more frequent episodes of hypoglycaemia and less frequent blood glucose monitoring.

Employment

 Key points

◆ Most people find that the diagnosis of diabetes makes little or no difference to their ability to work.

◆ There are some occupations, e.g. armed forces, emergency forces, and pilots, which exclude people with diabetes.

◆ People with diabetes are entitled to the benefit of the Disability Discrimination Act 1995.

◆ Shift workers may find that they have to make adjustments to their medication and lifestyle to maintain diabetes control.

I've got a niece now who's a diabetic in the States, and she's done everything that she wanted to do: she got a university education, she works. And I can remember writing to her at the time she was diagnosed at fifteen, and saying 'Jenny, you can do anything you want to do, don't let it stop you'.

Grace   type 1 diabetes

A diagnosis of diabetes may have implications for certain areas of employment, especially if treated by insulin. However, for most people, having diabetes does not make a difference to their ability to work.

Some occupations may involve some element of risk such as working with heavy machinery. Although people with diabetes are not prevented from these jobs, an employer may have to consider aspects such as physical fitness and frequency of hypoglycaemia when thinking of employing the person with diabetes.

There are currently limitations to recruitment in the following occupations for people with insulin-treated diabetes:

- Armed forces and Merchant Navy.

- Police and ambulance service.

- Airline pilot, air traffic control and, on some airlines, cabin crew.

- Driving LGVs or PCVs.

- Train driver.

- Prison service.

- Working offshore, e.g. on oil rigs, aboard cruise liners, regardless of the nature of the job.

- Fire fighters, if newly diagnosed.

Diabetes and the Disability Discrimination Act

Most application forms will ask if a potential employee has a disability. While many people with diabetes do not consider themselves disabled, they do have the protection of the Disability Discrimination Act (DDA) 1995. This means that a potential employer cannot use the fact that a person has diabetes to discriminate against them.

Employers are legally responsible for ensuring that discrimination does not occur in the workplace. This includes the need to make reasonable adjustments for people with disabilities. It is unlawful to discriminate against disabled people by treating disabled employees less favourably for a reason related to their disability without justification.

❓ FAQ

What may my employer have concerns about?

Some or all of the following may be of concern to a potential employer

◆ Is your diabetes well controlled?

◆ How are hypos managed?

◆ Is there any evidence of complications that may affect your ability to work?

What do I have to tell my employer?

It is up to you how much you tell your employer. However, if it affects your job it may be useful to talk to your employer especially if you need 'reasonable adjustments' to be made. These may be adjustments that allow time away from the workplace to:

◆ Blood test, snack, or inject insulin.

◆ Attend appointments with a healthcare professional.

If you choose not tell your employer that you have diabetes, and it then affects how you work, your employer is not under any obligation to make reasonable adjustments.

Shift work and diabetes

Shift work often causes difficulties with blood glucose control. Several aspects of shift work may affect how diabetes is managed. These include:

◆ Mealtimes that are often changed with rotating shifts.

◆ Differing sleep patterns.

◆ Differing levels of activity at different times of the day.

These changes in routine may result in difficulties with time and dose of both insulin injections and oral hypoglycaemic tablets. It may be useful to think about the following when planning shift work:

◆   Testing and recording blood glucose levels in order to determine any patterns, especially before and after eating.

◆   Planning meals and snacks during working hours.

◆   Dose and timing of medication.

Working with a health professional to plan appropriate and manageable medication regimens will mean that shift work and diabetes can be managed.

Travel

> ### ➲ Key points
>
> ◆   Different modes of transport will require different considerations and this will depend on diabetes treatment.
>
> ◆   Careful planning before any long trip or holiday may help prevent any problems related to diabetes.
>
> ◆   There may be need for some identification, especially if travelling by air.
>
> ◆   It is advisable to take out travel insurance that will cover any illness that occurs as a result of diabetes.

> I travel around the world on holidays, and with sensible precautions that's no problem whatsoever.
>
> Gillian   type 1 diabetes

For the person with diabetes, planning a long journey or a trip for business or holiday may require some extra preparation. Aspects such as how long the journey will be and how much time will be spent away from home will be important considerations.

Planning a journey

How long is the journey?

Careful preparation for any journey is important for the person with diabetes as it may prevent any untoward events, especially if there are problems with transport or delays. Here are some things to think about.

	Diabetes treated with insulin or sulphonylureas (e.g. gliclazide)	Other oral hypoglycaemic tablets (e.g. metformin)
A short journey, e.g. a commute to work or driving to the shops	Carry usual treatment for hypoglycaemia and medication as appropriate	No special consideration needed
Longer journey, e.g. travelling longer distances for holiday or business	Take twice as much medication, blood glucose testing equipment and hypoglycaemia treatment as may be needed	Take twice as much medication as may be needed and, if testing for blood glucose levels, take twice as much equipment as may be needed

How are you travelling?

The mode of transport will have a bearing on the preparation that may be required. For example, trains often have buffet cars, and food or snacks can be purchased en route. A long journey by coach, on the other hand, may require a packed lunch or snacks. Those whose diabetes is treated by insulin or sulphonylurea tablets, and those who perform blood tests regularly may find that more planning is required.

Diabetes treatment will have a bearing on the preparation that may be required. Metformin does not usually give rise to hypoglycaemia when taken alone, whereas insulin treatment may need to be tailored to the circumstances of the journey.

Travelling by car

If using insulin or sulphonyureas to treat diabetes, the driver must test blood glucose levels before setting off. Blood glucose levels below 5 mmol/l require treatment with extra carbohydrate and the journey should be delayed until levels return to more than 5 mmol/l. If the journey is a long one, then it is recommended that the driver stops every 2 hours, checks blood glucose levels and treats as necessary.

Travelling by public transport

If using insulin or sulphonyureas to treat diabetes it is recommended that any medication and treatment for hypoglycaemia is carried in hand luggage. It may be useful to carry some carbohydrate-based snacks in case of delays and do not rely on the availability of restaurants, cafes, or buffet cars on trains.

Travelling by air

Travelling by air will mean that some preparation is required for the person with diabetes, particularly if carrying insulin and blood glucose testing equipment. The following checklist may be useful when planning an air journey.

◆ Arrange to have some identification that you can carry stating you have diabetes. If treated with insulin and travelling by air, arrange to have a letter from your GP or hospital diabetes team, with a contact name, telephone number and address, stating you have diabetes and confirming the need to carry needles and syringes. For a nominal fee, Diabetes UK provide an Insulin Users ID card which may be useful when travelling through airport security.

◆ If not treated by insulin but using blood-testing equipment, it may be useful to have a letter from your GP stating that you have diabetes and are required to blood test regularly.

◆ Take twice as much medication, equipment, and any treatment for hypoglycaemia than may be needed and carry them in hand luggage so that they are easily accessible. Always place them in a clear plastic bag for easy inspection.

◆ If insulin is put in the main hold of an aircraft, the insulin will freeze, which means it will no longer be active and will not be suitable for use. If travelling for long periods, consider a cool bag for storing insulin.

◆ Carry blood-testing equipment in hand luggage, as frequent blood glucose testing may be required, especially on long journeys.

◆ Carry extra carbohydrate in hand luggage to allow for any delays during travel.

❓ FAQ

I have type 1 diabetes and am travelling from Land's End to John O'Groats by coach and then staying there for a week. What do I need to take with me?

◆ For a holiday like this, it will be important to make sure that you have enough insulin and to carry it in your hand luggage.

◆ Take some extra carbohydrate in case of any delays during the journey.

◆ Make sure that you have any treatment for hypoglycaemia easily to hand.

◆ Make sure you have enough blood-testing equipment with you.

Planning a holiday or business trip

When planning a longer trip either for business or holiday, it may be important to consider the following:

◆ Preparation for the trip.

◆ How to manage medication and travel to different time zones.

◆ The climate at the destination.

◆ Food and drink.

◆ Health and insurance.

Before the journey

Careful planning may avoid problems as a result of diabetes during any long break away from home. It may be useful to talk to a healthcare professional before the journey, especially if there are current health concerns or if any vaccinations are needed. The following may be a useful checklist of things to consider before travelling.

Checklist

◆ If arranging vaccinations, book them well in advance of travel, to allow management of any side effects should they occur.

◆ If travelling in Europe, obtain the European Health Insurance Card (EHIC), which allows access to free medical attention in EU countries.

- Arrange adequate travel insurance and inform the insurance company that you have diabetes. Not all insurance companies will provide cover for treatment of diabetes-related illnesses, so it will be important to make sure that your insurance cover is adequate.

- Arrange to have plentiful supplies of medication. It is useful to take at least double the amount of supplies than you would normally use in that time period.

Medication and time zones

In general, it is advised that management of medication during travel should be discussed with a health professional, who will advise on both timing and care of both oral hypoglycaemic agents and insulin. The timing of medication is important especially when passing through time zones, as days will be either shorter or longer depending on the direction of travel. During any long journey, it may be necessary to monitor blood glucose levels regularly and, if appropriate, ensure that hypoglycaemia treatment is available.

Climate

When travelling to places with either very hot or cold climate extremes, the following aspects of diabetes management should be considered:

Storage of medication: in hot climates, medication and blood-testing equipment should be kept cool and out of direct sunlight, and in cold climates should be protected from freezing.

Blood glucose control: in a hot climate, blood glucose levels may fall and in a cold climate blood glucose levels may rise. It will be important to test regularly and adjust medication as advised.

Blood glucose testing: in cold climates it may be difficult to obtain blood from fingertips, so it may be advisable to wear gloves and to warm hands before testing. Variation in climate may also affect blood glucose meters and strips, and it may be useful to discuss the type of meter and strips in use with a healthcare professional before travel.

Food and drink

A change of diet while on holiday may be a concern for the person with diabetes, and it may be useful to consider the following:

- Most countries include carbohydrate in their diet, but it may be unfamiliar, e.g. couscous in North Africa, chapattis in Pakistan, noodles in Japan.

- Take usual precautions regarding food safety and drinking water.

◆ Regular blood glucose testing and adjustment of medication may be necessary to manage any changes in diet.

Changes in time zones, climate and food may lead to unpredictable blood glucose levels. Adjustment in medication may be necessary, but a relatively short period of erratic blood glucose results should not affect overall diabetes control.

Health and insurance
Illness on holiday

If ill on holiday it will be important for the person with diabetes to follow 'sick-day rules' (see Chapter 4). If an illness persists it may be necessary to contact a local doctor for treatment. As with any illness, it is important for the person with diabetes to continue taking their diabetes treatment (insulin, tablets, or both), even if solid foods are not tolerated.

Travel insurance

If travel insurance is required, it will be important to ensure that it covers diabetes-related conditions, the charges for replacement of insulin or other medication and equipment, and emergency transport home if needed. Always tell the insurer that diabetes is present as a pre-existing medical condition.

Psychosocial issues

Diabetes is traditionally regarded as a physical disease, and most advice concentrates on the medical management of diabetes; controlling blood glucose levels, monitoring weight, blood pressure and blood lipid levels, and adjusting medication and lifestyle to produce the best outcome for these plysical measurements. What is frequently overlooked are the complex psychosocial issues that are associated with the diagnosis and management of diabetes and its consequences. An overview of these issues is provided here.

Children

Young children with diabetes rely upon their adult carers to provide the majority of decisions affecting their day-to-day life and health. Their family or carers are responsible for the monitoring, medical treatment, and lifestyle changes that are necessary for the child's normal growth and development. This responsibility can lead to overdependency in children and overprotectiveness in parents. As children grow and develop, they spend less time at home and more at school or in the company of friends, and they begin to assume responsibility for their diabetes. Studies have shown that children with diabetes move through these stages more comfortably if they have a family-based model of care which is supported by a specialist multidisciplinary team.

Adolescents

Adolescence is a time of great change and development in physical, mental, and emotional terms. It can be very challenging for both the adolescent with diabetes and their parents and carers as they move from total dependence on others to supported independent self-management. Peer pressure is very powerful in influencing the way an adolescent chooses to lead their life, and this can have an enormous impact on self-care among adolescents with diabetes. Traditionally, adolescence is the time for experimentation with food, alcohol, drugs, and sex, and all these can affect diabetes management. Research has shown that adolescents with diabetes who receive support and advice from their parents and carers, and who are not left to self-manage alone, do better that those in whom complete independence is encouraged.

Adults

The majority of adults are expected to provide their own day-to-day management of diabetes with all that this entails—medication acceptance and adherence, managing lifestyle factors such as diet and exercise, and monitoring glucose levels. Many people with diabetes report feeling 'burnt-out' by the pressures of managing diabetes, and it has been reported that people with diabetes are more likely to suffer from depression and emotional distress. This emotional distress is associated with poor quality of life and affects people's ability to care for themselves and their diabetes. It is advised that those who feel that they have emotional distress related to diabetes should discuss this with their healthcare professional and, if necessary, be referred to a behavioural or psychosocial specialist.

. . . my time for depression is when I'm on my own at night. I pretend a lot, because I feel I have to, because if I went around acting the way I feel sometimes, everybody would disown me, nobody would talk to me.

Shirley   type 2 diabetes

There are behavioural strategies that can be utilized to reduce the burden of diabetes distress, and research has shown that these can be effective in people with diabetes. Some people find that they benefit from prescribed medication if they are depressed.

Managing diabetes stress

Many people report that they find managing diabetes very stressful and that it has an effect on quality of life. It may be helpful to discuss issues around managing diabetes with a member of the healthcare team. There are behavioural strategies that can be used to help reduce the stress you are feeling; there is a brief description below of some of these.

◆ Cognitive behavioural therapy. This is a process encouraging identification of any negative, unrealistic thoughts (e.g. 'I can never do anything right so there's no point in trying') and helps to replace them with more positive realistic thoughts about the ability to manage diabetes (e.g. 'Sometimes it's hard to eat the right kinds of foods, but most of the time I manage').

◆ Behavioural interventions. These include a wide variety of strategies including goal-setting, motivational interviewing, problem-solving, self-monitoring, relapse prevention, and finding social support. Many health professionals receive training in these techniques and may be able to offer support in applying them in practice.

◆ The 5C intervention. This has been developed by American psychologists and uses a step-by-step approach for the five major steps supporting behaviour change. These five steps are:

1. Constructing a definition of a particular problem.

2. Collaborative goal-setting.

3. Collaborative problem-solving.

4. Contracting for change.

5. Continuing support.

All these approaches require some specialist training, but in many areas there are members of the healthcare team who have received the necessary training and may be able to offer support. In some areas, it is possible to refer people with diabetes to psychologists who have a specialist interest in diabetes.

Pregnancy

➲ Key points

◆ By taking care, a woman with diabetes can have a 'normal' pregnancy.

◆ It is important for mother and baby that diabetes control is as good as possible *before* becoming pregnant.

◆ Women with type 2 diabetes will need to stop oral medications and change to insulin ideally before becoming pregnant.

◆ During pregnancy even tighter control is required (i.e. more frequent testing and target blood glucose 6 mmol/l) to reduce chances of complications.

> Some people say you shouldn't get pregnant if you have diabetes, others say it is not a problem. I just want to know if the baby will be okay.

It is true to say that pregnancy in a person with diabetes is more complicated, but there is no reason, with the proper precautions, why it cannot proceed just as a pregnancy without diabetes. The precautions that are needed depend on the type of diabetes a person has. There are three types of diabetes in pregnancy:

1. **Type 1 diabetes that was present before conception**—insulin should be continued but the dose may well be increased during pregnancy.

2. **Type 2 diabetes that was present before conception**—the tablets need to be stopped and insulin started as soon as a woman finds out she is pregnant. Insulin can usually be stopped and tablets restarted once the baby is born and has stopped breastfeeding.

3. **Gestational diabetes**—is diagnosed first during pregnancy and usually comes on in the second half of pregnancy. It may be controlled with diet alone; if not, insulin will be started. This can usually stop once the baby is born; however, gestational diabetes is often a sign that type 2 diabetes will develop later in a woman's life.

Preparing for pregnancy

General advice

Probably one of the most prudent precautions a woman with diabetes can take is actually seeking advice from a healthcare professional *before* she conceives. The most important concern is to have good control at the time of conception: this greatly reduces the chance of miscarriage and congenital malformations, which are the result of poor glucose control at the time of conception or just after, between 5 and 9 weeks when a woman may not even know she is pregnant. *Ideally HbA1c should be stable and within target for 3 months before conception.*

It is also advisable to have eyes and kidneys checked as a baseline for comparison during pregnancy.

Folic acid tablets should be started a month before conception, as with women who do not have diabetes, to reduce the risk of having a baby with spina bifida.

Finally, as with women who do not have diabetes, it is advisable to stop smoking and drinking alcohol whilst trying to conceive, and definitely after becoming pregnant.

Type 1 diabetes

A woman suffering with recurrent DKA should not try to conceive, as ketones can also damage the foetus.

Type 2 diabetes

A woman with diabetes should stop any drugs that could harm a foetus, including all oral tablets for type 2 diabetes (and insulin will be required in their place).

If a woman is significantly overweight, this increases risk of high blood pressure during the pregnancy, and a target weight will often be suggested before a woman should get pregnant.

Managing diabetes during pregnancy

General advice for all types of diabetes

◆ It is advisable to continue folic acid for the first 12 weeks of pregnancy.

◆ It is important to have regular scans initially at 10–12 weeks to look for congenital abnormalities and to confirm dates. Repeat scans to check for excessive growth/macrosomia at 18–20 weeks, 28 weeks, 32 weeks, and 36 weeks are recommended.

◆ More frequent blood testing is also recommended, with a tighter target around 6 mmol/l.

Type 1 diabetes

Women with **type 1 diabetes** can require 2–3 times the usual dose of insulin. This is because during pregnancy several hormones contribute to increasing the blood glucose levels available for the foetus. Towards the end of pregnancy, and certainly after the baby is born, insulin requirements drop right down again.

It is even more important to eat regularly, three meals a day and a bedtime snack, to avoid a long fast overnight which may prompt ketoacidosis. It is worthwhile consulting a dietician for some specific tips about your daily intake and what it should consist of.

❓ FAQ

Will pregnancy make any difference to my eyes?

If a woman has severe retinopathy before pregnancy this may deteriorate during pregnancy. It will be monitored regularly during the pregnancy, and usually returns to the previous state once the baby is born.

Will pregnancy make any difference to my kidney failure?

If a woman has severe nephropathy (or diabetes affecting the kidney) there is a chance of high blood pressure or toxaemia in pregnancy. These can be treated, but it is worth having a discussion with a specialist in diabetes and pregnancy about the risks to the long-term health of the mother.

Type 2 diabetes

In overweight women, less weight should be gained during the pregnancy. Insulin is almost always required and therefore necessitates more frequent blood glucose testing and care to avoid both hypoglycaemia and hyperglycaemia.

Gestational diabetes

This is picked up by sugar present in the urine. This prompts a blood test for raised glucose, and if this is high the woman will have an oral glucose tolerance test. If a person has had gestational diabetes in a previous pregnancy she is treated as though she has gestational diabetes in all future pregnancies.

Managing hypoglycaemia during pregnancy

Hypoglycaemia can occur more frequently in pregnancy. This is often due to striving to achieve tighter control. In addition, there is also possible loss of usual warning signs in the later part of pregnancy. Therefore, it is really crucial first to test more frequently and secondly to eat regularly with enough carbohydrate in the diet. It can be really helpful to seek advice from a dietician at the beginning of pregnancy.

Complications: miscarriage and congenital malformations

❓ FAQ

Am I more likely to have a miscarriage?

Around 16% of apparently normal pregnancies without diabetes are lost through spontaneous miscarriage. In well-controlled diabetes, the miscarriage rate does not appear to be any higher than in women without diabetes.

Will having diabetes affect my baby?

The chance of major congenital malformation is 2–3% without diabetes but rises to 7–13% with poorly controlled diabetes. With good diabetes care before conception, this risk can come down to 1–5%.

Macrosomia is the technical term for an abnormally large baby. This can cause complications at birth, increasing risk of a Caesarean section. It occurs when a mother's glucose is high during pregnancy, as this sugar passes through the placenta to the foetus. With persistently high levels of glucose, the foetus' own pancreas produces a lot of insulin which does not pass back across the placenta to the maternal blood. The high levels of insulin and sugar in the foetal blood cause fat to develop and the baby is born large. If the mother's diabetes is well controlled, this cycle does not occur.

Labour and delivery

The chance of a long labour and assisted delivery (forceps, vonteuse, or Caesarean section) is increased with a large baby, especially if born to a small mother. There is also a risk of **neonatal hypoglycaemia** in the first few days. This is because the foetus makes a lot of insulin to handle the high maternal glucose which is then suddenly cut off at birth. As the high level of foetal insulin hangs around for a while, there can be hypoglycaemia in the first 4–6 hours after delivery. Therefore, it will be necessary to do hourly blood glucose levels on the baby after birth.

If the baby is premature, it can suffer with low calcium or magnesium which can cause jitteriness or seizures. This can be replaced until the baby makes enough for itself. Respiratory distress is also a risk linked to prematurity but responds well to treatment and tends not to occur with good prenatal care. Jaundice and bowel obstruction can occur, but most often these resolve spontaneously.

If there were very high levels of glucose or ketones during pregnancy, a baby may show lower intelligence which is not apparent at birth but may be noted later. If a baby is very large, this weight is generally lost in the first year but it can be predisposed to obesity later in childhood.

Although the list of complications is long, with good pre-conception control, which continues through the pregnancy, there is no reason why the risk of any complication should not be kept very low and proceed in the same way as a pregnancy without diabetes.

After the delivery and looking after a newborn

Insulin requirements can drop by 50% immediately after delivery. Usually pre-pregnancy regimes are returned to once the woman is eating normally, but in the first 24 hours after delivery insulin requirements can be particularly low.

There are no reasons why a mother with diabetes cannot breastfeed. There is increased potential for hypoglycaemia, and extra carbohydrate snacks for the mother are often needed as well as a 20–25% reduction in pre-conception insulin requirements. Oral diabetes medications should not be restarted until breastfeeding has stopped.

? FAQ

If the father is the one with diabetes, does this cause any risk to the baby?

In terms of congenital malformations and miscarriage, no, the baby should develop normally. The risks only apply if the mother has the diabetes as it is the environment that the foetus develops in that can potentially cause problems.

In terms of inheritance of diabetes, there is an increased risk of diabetes developing in the child of either parent with diabetes.

6

Long-term complications of diabetes

Introduction

Diabetes is characterized by having a higher than normal blood glucose concentration in the body. When insulin was discovered in 1922, it was thought for a while that this would be a complete cure—that taking insulin and avoiding very high or very low glucose levels would be all that would be required. However, it became apparent, over the years, that having higher glucose over a long period of time could lead to stiffening of the blood vessels, and a consequent reduction in oxygen and nutrients to the tissues. This could happen to the large blood vessels (macrovascular) to the heart, brain and legs, and to the small vessel networks (microvascular) such as those to the eyes, kidneys, and nerves. These effects cause the so-called 'long-term complications' of diabetes, and much of the routine care in diabetes is directed towards prevention of these complications. They are heart attacks, stroke, poor circulation in the legs, problems with the back of the eyes (retinopathy), problems with kidney disease (nephropathy), and problems in the nerves, especially, but not exclusively, of the lower limb (neuropathy).

Heart attacks and stroke

Atherosclerosis

Atherosclerosis is a particular complication of large vessels. As well as the vessels becoming stiff, deposits of fat and fibrous tissue in their walls can build up, and sometimes lead to a breakage or rupture of the vessel. Atherosclerosis is the main cause of the narrowing or 'furring up' of the arteries, with the formation of thickened areas known as 'plaques'. Atherosclerosis can be influenced and accelerated by a rise in cholesterol levels—as certain types of fat form a major part of the plaques. Therefore, there has been a particular concentration on ways in which these processes can be slowed: reducing cholesterol, stopping smoking, reducing blood pressure, and adopting a healthy lifestyle, including adequate intake of fruit and vegetables, and regular exercise. All these aim to reduce or slow the damaging processes.

Assessing cardiovascular risk

Many research studies have looked at identifying particular elements within a person's lifestyle and physique that might increase their risk of atherosclerosis affecting vessels throughout the body, known also as cardiovascular disease. Recognition of these allows those people at high cardiovascular risk to be identified earlier and treated sooner. Some of these factors cannot be influenced, such as incidence increasing with age, and men being more susceptible at all ages than women. This last effect is partly reflected by a difference in fat distribution between the two sexes. In women, storage of fat tends to be in the thigh and buttock area, while men tend to expand their waist measurement as they put on weight in middle age. Some have described this as a pear-shape of women and an apple-shape of men. It can be assessed by waist measurement, which is emerging as one of the best simple markers of cardiovascular risk as it gives an indication of fat distribution. We also know that certain races have an increased cardiovascular risk.

Can cardiovascular disease risk be improved?
Modifiable cardiovascular risk factors

Large trials have shown that risks can be reduced. Some risks relate to lifestyle, and some to genetic factors that can best be altered by drugs.

Blood glucose. It follows logically from understanding the causes of stiffening arteries that blood glucose needs to be carefully controlled. That means

Table 6.1 Identified cardiovascular risk factors

Modifiable	Non-modifiable
Blood glucose	Gender
Smoking	Age
Blood pressure	Ethnic origin
Blood lipids (cholesterol, etc.)	
Weight/waist measurement	
Diet	
Exercise	

getting the values to as near normal as possible, but it is no use doing this if it means that there are periods where the levels are too low. That causes hypoglycaemia (see Chapter 4).

Smoking. This is a very addictive habit which carries an increased risk of cancer and heart disease especially. The risks of smoking are astonishingly high. Smoking-related illness will kill one out of every two people who smoke, or, put another way, takes 10 years of life expectancy off everyone who smokes.

> It seems extraordinary that cigarette smoking is so dangerous that it is a greater risk than all the other risks put together. It seems ridiculous, when you put it like this, but it is true.
>
> Sir Richard Doll   www.OxHa.com

There are now many options available to help in giving up smoking, which is especially important in people with diabetes. Most general practices will have a stop-smoking programme, and nicotine replacement using patches or other methods of administration can be of particular help. It is also worth noting that it is very difficult to give up smoking if someone else in the household continues to smoke—the availability of the cigarettes and the temptation together can be hard to resist. So stopping smoking should ideally be a household decision—after all everyone will gain in health and in financial terms, and everyone can support each other in their resolve.

Blood pressure. One of the signs of stiffening of blood vessels, especially arteries, is an increase in blood pressure. High blood pressure can cause sudden damage such as strokes—where the pressure may burst a blood vessel in the brain. It can also damage organs slowly over the years, and this is especially true of the kidney, where one of the signs may be a small leakage of proteins detectable in the urine. High blood pressure, in itself, may cause no symptoms at all, so having blood pressure checked regularly is important. Recent research suggests that even lowering blood pressure below what can be regarded as normal can be helpful in reducing risks.

Blood fats. There are several different types of fat (lipid) found in the blood, the most important ones being cholesterol and triglycerides. Cholesterol is the fat that most people know about, and it is essential for creating and maintaining the membranes that surround every cell in the body. It is a constituent of the brain and of some of the body's chemical messengers (hormones). Often the total blood cholesterol is measured, and this gives some guide as to whether treatment is necessary. Often, however, separate fractions of cholesterol are measured as some cholesterol can be regarded as 'good' and some not! The lay term 'good cholesterol' refers to HDL (high-density lipoprotein) and it is this cholesterol that one would, appropriately, like to be **high**, whereas LDL (low-density lipoprotein) is most strongly associated with an increased risk of cardiovascular disease, and this should be kept as **low** as possible. One would like, ideally, to have an HDL above 1.2 mmol, and some people have values as high as 2.4 or more. They have relative protection against heart disease. One would like the LDL to be 3.5 or lower. How can we put these figures together into a form that takes account of both? The answer is that often a ratio of total cholesterol divided by HDL is used, and ratios of 4 or below are currently being advised.

Then there is another fat, 'triglyceride', which provides a very useful high energy store. However, triglyceride must first be transported from the gut to the various organs requiring an energy source (such as muscle) or energy store (body fat). High triglycerides increase the risk of atherosclerosis development, and the aim is to keep these in the normal range below about 1.5 mmol/l. Triglycerides can sometimes get to massively high levels, and levels of 30 mmol/l or more can occur. This needs prompt treatment.

Blood fats can be controlled by maintaining a healthy lifestyle, and medication called 'statins' if required.

Weight, body mass index, and waist measurement

Weight is easy to measure, and everyone has an some idea of what they 'should' weigh—though there is a tendency for this value to increase. Healthcare professionals like to have a measure that allows for the fact that everyone is a different height, and they use the body mass index (BMI). This can be calculated as weight (in kilograms) divided by height (in metres) and divided again by height (in metres). Mathematically this is expressed as W/H^2. This allows definitions that apply to the population. A BMI of 20–25 is normal, greater than 25–30 is overweight and greater than 30 is obese. Overweight is a risk for developing diabetes and is also frequently used as a measure of cardiovascular disease risk.

Waist measurement is a quick way of assessing the size of the abdomen, and this can then be used as a risk marker.

Cardiovascular risk factor reduction

- Blood glucose—as well controlled as individually possible, with minimal short-lived elevations, without resort to recurrent hypoglycaemia.

- Smoking—stop as soon as possible. Make use of support available. Get everyone in the household to stop together.

- Blood pressure—regular measurements to assess risk and medication may be useful in reducing high levels.

- Blood fats—aim for high, 'good' (HDL) and low, 'bad' (LDL) cholesterol and triglycerides. Medication may be useful in improving the profile.

- Weight/waist measurement—a useful marker, easy to monitor.

- Diet—healthy, balanced intake without excessive energy/calories (kcal) (see Chapter 2).

- Exercise—adequate physical activity (see Chapter 2).

Angina and heart attack (myocardial infarction)

The heart is the blood pump of the body, and in order to function needs a blood supply of its own to provide its muscle cells with oxygen and energy. There are three main blood vessels that supply the heart, and damage to or narrowing of any of these may produce symptoms of oxygen starvation in the heart muscle. This is painful and is called angina. If the blood flow is severely restricted or reduced for a longer period of time, parts of the heart muscle may become irreversibly damaged, known as a heart attack (myocardial infarction or MI). If large areas of the heart are damaged, then the heart will beat irregularly or simply stop. Death will occur unless resuscitation can be promptly provided.

Angina often produces a temporary feeling of tightness in the chest, often described as a band-like or crushing pain. Cold weather, strong winds, eating a large meal, and physical exertion all increase the effort of the heart and therefore increase the blood demand, which increases the chances of angina. Heart attacks are usually associated with more severe chest pain, breathlessness, pallor, and sweating, and the pain may spread to the neck, jaw, or down the left arm. However, in those who have diabetes, angina and even heart attacks may not be associated with the typical painful symptoms. The result may be a feeling of general unwellness with few clues as to the underlying reason.

And I was diagnosed with angina, but no actual pain, just breathless and had to sit down a bit and carried on again afterwards. It's funny—angina without pain; I can't understand it, but . . . Even a heart attack and the stroke, there was no pain whatsoever.

Richard

Early admission to hospital after the sudden onset of a heart attack allows treatment, and the earlier the admission the more likely it is that successful treatment can be given. Medications exist to 'dissolve' clots in the blood vessels supplying the heart (known as clot busters). This does not take the underlying narrowing away completely but it often improves symptoms quickly and reduces the amount of damage to the heart muscle. It also allows time for further investigations and treatment. This may include visualizing the structure of the blood vessels supplying the heart and the extent of the narrowing using X-ray techniques (angiography). Introducing a small tube or 'stent' through a large leg vessel and then into the heart's blood supply arteries (angioplasty) may be suggested in order to reduce the risk of a future heart attack.

Strokes and mini-strokes

Atherosclerosis may cause narrowing inside two important vessels—the large *carotid* arteries in the neck that carry most blood to the brain. This progressive narrowing process can eventually interrupt or reduce the blood supply to the brain, and give rise to strokes (sometimes called cerebrovascular accidents or *CVAs*) or mini-strokes (transient ischaemic attacks or TIAs).

Transient ischaemic attacks

Transient ischaemic attacks (TIAs) are temporary interruptions of blood supply to part of the brain. They can produce various symptoms, including weakness or numbness in the arms, face, or legs, difficulty in swallowing, talking, co-ordination or thought, and alterations in vision. The symptoms can be severe, but may last only a few minutes, and all these features completely disappear within 24 hours and leave no residual effect. TIAs indicate the presence of atherosclerosis affecting the blood supply to the brain. This can have the potential to continue and for the interruption to progress, resulting in damage and a more permanent stroke. About 10% of strokes are preceded by TIAs, so it is a strong warning sign of potential future risk. The symptoms of a TIA should be discussed urgently with healthcare professionals. Action should be taken early and urgently, and those with such events should be referred for medical attention immediately. Control of blood pressure, aspirin treatment, scanning, and radiological investigations may all be indicated.

Stroke (cerebrovascular accident or CVA)

A stroke is the result of permanent damage to areas of the brain by a reduction or stoppage in blood supply. Strokes occur when arteries to active brain tissue become blocked or rupture (haemorrhage), reducing the oxygen supply to that part of the brain and resulting in death of the brain cells within a few minutes if the blood supply is not reinstated. Even if these symptoms are temporary, as in TIAs, it is important to take them seriously as a warning sign of vessel disease, and a potential heralding symptom for more permanent damage.

Strokes and TIAs may present in many different ways, with sudden onset of any of the following symptoms. The differentiation between the two forms of cerebrovascular disease lies in the duration of the effects.

Symptoms of strokes and TIAs

- Severe headache.

- Numbness or weakness of the face, arm or leg, particularly if on one side of the body only.

- Difficulty in talking or swallowing.

- Confusion or difficulty in understanding.

- Change or loss of vision in one or both eyes.

- Dizziness or difficulty in co-ordination.

Diagnosis

The diagnosis of stroke or TIA relies on recognition of the symptoms (aspects that patients describe) and signs (changes found on examination). A full history and examination is followed by investigations, often including a scan of the brain to visualize directly any changes in appearance of local areas of the brain. This may be followed by an ultrasound investigation of the carotid arteries in the neck and maybe further investigations looking for the exact cause and location of narrowing in the arteries higher up in the head, using dye injections and radiological imaging techniques.

Treatment

'Clot buster drugs', as in the case of heart attacks, can be used to dissolve clots causing strokes. The effectiveness of this treatment relies on the drug being given very soon after the event in order to reduce the overall area of residual tissue damage, and so the occurrence of a stroke is a medical emergency. Surgery to remove atherosclerotic plaques from the carotid arteries in the neck may also be considered, or a stent may be put in place to open the carotid arteries. Rehabilitation from the effects of the stroke includes multidisciplinary help from physiotherapists, occupational therapists, and speech therapists in some cases, as well as counselling, and review and reduction of major risk factors to prevent any recurrence.

Prevention

The risk of stroke can be reduced by recognition of risk factors increasing the chances of such a condition. Control of high blood pressure is a particularly important factor in risk reduction, and recognition of a family history of previous stroke in first-degree relatives, particularly if they occur at a young age (less than 50 years), can help to identify further those at increased risk. Diabetes increases the risk of stroke by accelerating the processes of atherosclerosis, or narrowing of the arteries. Maintaining good glycaemic control is known to reduce this risk, as is control of blood lipids (cholesterol in particular), regular physical activity, and being a non-smoker. As with cardiovascular disease, the presence of two or more factors in combination results in a multiplication of the risk rather than just simple addition. So identification and advice or medication for *each* individual risk factor is important.

Risk factors for TIAs and strokes

- Diabetes.

- High blood pressure.

- High blood cholesterol levels.

- Smoking.

- Previous stroke, TIA, heart attack, or peripheral vascular disease.

- Family history of stroke or TIAs.

Peripheral vascular disease

The other type of macrovascular disease affecting the general population, with an increased risk in those people with diabetes, is known as peripheral vascular disease. This refers to its effects on the blood supply to 'peripheral' tissues, furthest from the central heart pump, and usually specifically means foot and leg disease. The legs are supplied with blood from a large central vessel in the abdomen which splits in two to provide blood to both limbs. The vessels then continue down the length of the legs, getting progressively smaller and smaller, as the leg become thinner, into the foot. The smaller the vessel, the easier it is to block the blood flow by atherosclerosis or development of a clot.

Symptoms

Initial symptoms of impaired blood supply to one or both legs include cramping in the muscles, particularly in the calves, and a burning feeling (called 'claudication'—see page 140 for more details on this). Reduced blood supply means the muscles work less effectively and walking can be limited. Any healing or repair processes require a healthy blood supply. An injury to an area of poor blood supply is likely to heal less quickly and may not completely heal. This increases the chance of infection in the wound and potentially the underlying bone. Bone has a relatively poor blood supply, making the delivery of antibiotics particularly difficult, and infection of bony structures (osteomyelitis) can be very difficult to treat.

Treatment

Exercise in the early stages of peripheral vascular disease increases the development and blood flow in these tributaries, and can improve symptoms. Apart from the benefit of good glycaemic control and general cardiovascular risk factor reduction (especially stopping smoking), it is possible in some cases to identify and unblock the narrowed artery. This requires inserting a thin tube into the top of the major leg vessel and first visualizing the inside of the vessel using dye and radiography imaging techniques (angiogram). If the narrowing is short and in an accessible position, it is sometimes possible to insert a thin stent into the vessel to open it out and return blood flow (angioplasty) (see page 146). Alternative treatment might include operative repair of the narrowed section by inserting another blood vessel in its place—usually a vein from the lower part of the leg that the body can manage well without (see page 149). Both of these treatments may solve the problem, but the solution may be temporary if re-narrowing occurs.

> They decided they could do the angioplasties, and I had one done in November and the other leg in January . . . I felt as if I'd got one leg that was lighter than the other, and when the other leg was done . . . we went walking, and I climbed up a steep sort of ladder-cum-staircase, and we walked round the island for hours, and it was like having a second life, you know, it really was wonderful.
>
> Erika

Preventative treatments in cardiovascular disease

Some medications are taken by people to reduce the possible risk of heart attacks, strokes, or peripheral vascular disease in the future if they have been identified as 'at risk'. Having a diagnosis of diabetes does increase your potential risk of cardiovascular disease, and so these forms of medication are commonly used in people with diabetes. Many people start these medications when they are fit and healthy, with no signs of cardiovascular disease, in the hope of preventing any complication occurring.

Aspirin

A small dose of aspirin (75 mg or a quarter of a standard aspirin tablet) in people over the age of 50 years has been shown to be effective in reducing the 'stickiness' of blood. A possible side effect of taking regular aspirin is indigestion—a burning or acid sensation in the stomach. If this occurs it is important to discuss these symptoms with a doctor.

Statins

This group of medications can be very useful in reducing blood fats. Possible side effects with statins include muscular aches and pains. These only occur in a small proportion of people taking the medication, but any possible symptoms are worth discussing with a doctor for advice.

Blood pressure controlling agents

Several different groups of medication fall into this category, each with differing side effects and individual effectiveness. The need to control blood pressure to an acceptable level may well require combination of several different types of blood pressure medication.

Table 6.2 Cardiovascular disease prevention

Medication	Action	Possible side effects
Aspirin (75 mg or a quarter of a standard aspirin tablet)	Reduces the 'stickiness' of the blood. An increased stickiness means a risk of clots forming inside vessels, particularly if already narrowed by atherosclerosis	Indigestion
Clopidogrel	A clot-reducing drug that can be particularly helpful in peripheral vascular disease treatment	
Statins	Can be very useful in reducing a person's cholesterol	Muscular aches and pains

(continued)

Table 6.2 Cardiovascular disease prevention *(continued)*

Medication	Action	Possible side effects
ACE inhibitors	These act by reducing the activity of a chemical messenger involved in controlling blood pressure, and they can also help protect the kidneys from damage due to diabetes	Dry cough in around 10% of people. If this occurs, medication can be changed to a similar type of drug without this side effect.

Exercise is also beneficial in almost all situations, in health and in preventing disease. Moderation and a gentle start are encouraged to make sure no complications occur from the effects of exercise. A healthy diet and controlling weight also have an important effect on cardiovascular risk.

Feet—neuropathy

Introduction

Foot problems are associated with diabetes because diabetes can cause nerve damage (peripheral neuropathy) and poor circulation (peripheral vascular disease). This, together with a reduced ability to fight infection, makes minor injury, or trauma and ulceration, a particular problem. However, feet ulcerations only occur in a few of those with diabetes, and even in those who do get problems, prompt action and good podiatry (or chiropody) will prevent any serious outcome.

Nerve damage

> I noticed some blood on the floor when I took off my shoe and found a drawing pin embedded through my sock into my foot . . . It did not hurt!
>
> Dave   type 2 diabetes for past 12 years

Nerve damage or neuropathy can occur in up to 50% of people with diabetes, leading to diabetic neuropathy, affecting three types of nerve.

Sensory nerve damage

First, sensory nerves can be affected. These nerves provide the body with information about the outside world: temperature, pain, pressure, vibration, or position of the foot. A common problem in those with sensory nerve loss is the failure to perceive that the bath water is too hot, or that a shoe is rubbing on the skin. This form of neuropathy begins at the extremities (the tips of the toes, or, much less commonly, the fingers)—which has been termed 'the periphery'. So 'peripheral sensory neuropathy' begins with, perhaps, a tiny loss of sensation at the big toe and then may progress to involve the foot or the foot and the ankle together. The shape is like a sock, and for this reason it is termed a 'stocking distribution' of sensation loss.

Painful feet

Although some people with diabetes have reduced sensation, or numbness in their feet, others have painful neuropathy and complain of tightness, stiffness in the skin, heightened awareness of sensation (hyperaesthesiae), coldness, pins and needles (paraesthesiae), walking on stones (metatarsalgia), burning sensations and unpleasant sensation (allodynia), particularly at night with the feet feeling too hot. Sometimes the touch of the bedclothes causes irritation. This is due to normal stimulus, such as touch, being incorrectly transmitted by damaged nerves to the brain as painful stimuli.

Painless painful feet

Some people with diabetes may have nerve damage that fails to detect harmful sensations such as the pain of standing on a nail, but transmits pain from harmless stimuli such as the feel of clothes, socks, and bedsheets as pain.

Balance

My balance does not seem so good lately. I have to hold on to things sometimes, or I feel as though I will fall.

Hazel   type 1 diabetes

Peripheral neuropathy may also lead to poor feedback from skin, bones, and joints in the feet (proprioception), leading to increasing problems with balance in some people with diabetes.

I keep on getting cracks around my heels. Sometimes they are deep and bleed.

Carol   type 2 diabetes

Autonomic nerve damage

A second set of nerves that can be damaged in diabetes are the 'autonomic' nerves, which control functions that are not under our conscious control. So, for example, the control of sweating can be affected, resulting in dry skin and the loss of its elasticity. This can lead to splitting, or cracking.

Autonomic neuropathy also affects the blood flow in the foot, which travels through large supply blood vessels (arteries) into smaller vessels (arterioles) and then into a mesh of tiny vessels (capillaries) where oxygen and other products are delivered to the tissues of the foot. Waste products and carbon dioxide are collected from the tissues by the same capillaries into the returning small blood vessels (venules), and then to larger returning blood vessels, the veins.

> My toes seem to have changed shape: they are all curled up, and I seem to be walking on the tips now.
>
> Miles   type 2 diabetes

The foot also has shunts where blood travels from arteries to veins bypassing the capillaries. In those with autonomic nerve damage these shunts may remain open, resulting in a warmer swollen foot with bulging (dilated) veins that are easily seen on the top of the foot through the surface of the skin. As a result of this, the supply of blood to the tissues by the capillaries may be reduced, and this in turn may affect the body's ability to fight infection, or heal a wound.

Motor nerve damage

The third set of nerves that can be affected are the motor nerves, which control movement through muscles, and can lead to reduced function, wasting of muscles (atrophy), and an alteration in the shape of the foot, leading to deformity. Motor neuropathy can be isolated, but is often combined with a change in the sensations, and can often occur at the same time with a very painful fast onset of weakness in one or both legs. This 'amyotrophy' is relatively rare, but when it occurs it will need careful medication to control the pain and careful physiotherapy when the acute phase—typically several months—is passed.

Charcot foot

> I noticed that after missing the step last month I can no longer wear my shoes. I have to wear my boots now, but the foot does not hurt.
>
> Tom   type 2 diabetes

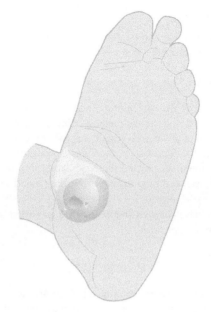

Figure 6.1 Charcot foot with ulcer.

Patients with peripheral neuropathy may develop a condition called Charcot foot after minor injury. The foot may become red and swollen and, if left untreated, may change shape due to the joints/bones in the foot becoming slowly fragmented. The integrity of the foot becomes destroyed and the arch may drop, causing abnormal pressure areas and secondary ulceration.

If this condition is noticed quickly and treated with offloading, by plaster casts or walkers, the active destructive phase of the condition will burn itself out over some months. If, during this time, the shape of the foot can be preserved, this will help to prevent ulceration in the future. It is therefore important to seek professional help quickly if there is a change in foot shape. Charcot feet are, however, rare. It is important to distinguish it from infection or a deep vein thrombosis.

Poor circulation

It is important to appreciate the difference between the peripheral circulatory system and the peripheral nervous system. The best analogy to understand the difference is that nerves are like electrical cables taking signals from the brain to the feet and the feet to the brain, whereas the peripheral circulation is like plumbing taking blood from the heart to the feet through arteries and returning it in another set of vessels called veins.

The prevalence of peripheral vascular disease in people with diabetes is somewhere between 15% and 30%, and it becomes more common with advancing age and with a long duration of diabetes.

> I get pain in my calf if I walk too far, especially if I go up a hill or up steps
>
> Geoff   type 1 diabetes

The normal large arteries in the lower limb gradually become narrower in diameter further down the leg. However, with diabetes, they may narrow further because of so-called arterial plaque (stenosis), or they may even become blocked (occluded). This poor circulation (ischaemia) may give rise to pain in the buttocks, thigh, calf, or foot, and the pain may be worse on activity. This can cause limping, and the condition is named after the first-century Roman emperor, Claudius, who limped: 'claudication' limits the walking distance of a person, who may need to stop while pain in the leg subsides.

Claudication can often be mild with few symptoms limited perhaps to numbness or tiredness of the legs. At this stage, the blood supply to the lower limb is likely to be adequate.

Intermittent claudication occurs with more serious blockages, and this shows itself with an inability to walk because of pain—usually in the calf or back of the legs. Interestingly it has been demonstrated that in order to stimulate more blood vessels to grow, one should continue to walk through the pain as much as possible.

With more serious restriction of the blood supply, patients may experience 'rest pain'. Rest pain can become intense and may need powerful painkillers.

With critical reduction in blood supply, the tissues will develop gangrene. This is similar to frost-bite, and will need very careful intervention to avoid disasters. Treatment for vascular disease that is this serious needs to be undertaken in a specialist or hospital setting. Vascular surgeons may be needed to rebuild the blood supply and, in cases of critical ischaemia, amputation may be the only life-saving procedure possible.

Infection

Those with diabetes are more prone to infection as high blood glucose levels impair the body's immune system and bacteria thrive on sugars. So it is common for foot ulcers to become seriously infected, and this infection may affect the soft tissue (cellulitis), or penetrate deep into the foot and infect the bones (osteomyelitis).

Ulceration

So what is a diabetic foot ulcer and why do foot ulcers occur?

The International Working Group on the Diabetic Foot (wounds section) defined a diabetic foot ulcer as an erosion of the epidermis (skin) below the ankle in a person with diabetes. The acronym Now Do Take Care can be used to explain the underlying nature of the development to foot ulceration:

Nerve damage to the feet

Deformity to the feet

Trauma or injury to the feet

Circulation is poor to the feet.

Important risk factors and how to assess them

Nerve damage

A doctor or podiatrist may screen for peripheral neuropathy using a tuning fork, or an electrical device called a neurothesiometer. Here a person's ability to sense vibration is being tested. Small hair-like monofilaments may be pressed on to the skin of the feet and are used to detect if normal light touch sensation is present. Sharp sensation may be tested with a sterile pin, or 'neurotip' placed on the skin. Knee and ankle jerks may be performed to test reflexes, and a history of sensations felt—numbness, burning, tingling sensations—may be elicited.

In some instances, patients may be referred for nerve conduction studies or further neurophysiological testing.

Poor circulation

The palpation of foot pulses remains an important feature of screening for peripheral vascular disease. A history of intermittent claudication (see above), walking distance, rest pain, and the measurement of blood pressure at the ankle (ankle brachial pressure index) may indicate that more detailed investigations be instigated. An ultrasound duplex scan, or a scan of the arteries after dye or contrast media is injected into the arteries of the lower limb (angiogram) may be recommended.

Infection

If a doctor, podiatrist, or nurse thinks that a foot they are examining has an infection, they may take a specimen of blood, or a swab, or tissue sample from an ulcer to determine the nature of infection and discover which type of bacteria are causing it. These samples may also be used to discover which antibiotics might be appropriate.

The diagnosis of a foot infection is made by observing any redness, discharge, swelling, increasing warmth, change in colour, smell, or pain. All these bring a suspicion of infection. Red lines from the foot travelling up the leg may indicate that the infection is spreading, and any flu- or fever-like symptoms may indicate that the infection is spreading in the blood supply around the body. Antibiotics are clearly going to be necessary under these latter circumstances and, once an infection has taken control in anything other than a small area, specialist or hospital treatment is really essential.

A suspicion of bone involvement may be assessed with plain X-rays or a magnetic resonance image (MRI). These are important procedures to assess how long, and sometimes of what type of, antibiotics should be administered.

Deformity

There is a wide range of foot shape in the general population, with deformity producing bunions (deformity of the big toe), minor toe abnormality (claw, hammer toes), flat feet (pes planus), or high arched feet (pes cavus).

However, in the neuropathic foot, because of muscle imbalance, deformity may take the form of a high arched foot, with forward and downward pressure causing the toes to be bent into a claw or hammer shape.

In some instances the normal tissue padding over the natural foot pads on the sole of the foot may be reduced. This also leads to increased foot pressure and the possibility of ulceration. All those with diabetes who have these risky shapes to their feet should be referred to a podiatrist for an assessment.

Having some degree of foot deformity will put a person with diabetes more at risk of developing an ulcer. This can happen suddenly, with a blister, or more slowly, with a corn or callus breaking down with the increased pressure. Neuropathy can exacerbate the situation because of the reduced pain sensation.

Corns and calluses

Deformity may lead to increased pressure and, over time, to diffuse thickening of the skin (epidermis)—in particular the top layer of the skin (stratum corneum).

143

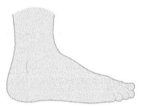

Figure 6.2 Flat foot.

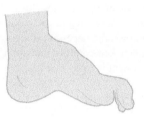

Figure 6.3 High arched foot.

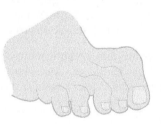

Figure 6.4 Clawed toes.

If the pressure is over a wide area, callus formation may occur. If the pressure is highly localized then a corn will form, producing a deeper formation of hard keratin, in turn causing more pressure. Those with corns or calluses should be referred to a podiatrist for assessment and treatment.

Ulceration

Having corns and calluses indicates that the feet are being traumatized. Over time the hard skin behaves like a foreign body and this reduces the elasticity of

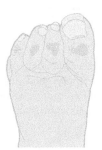

Figure 6.5 Bunion and clawing of toes, with corns forming.

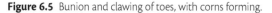

the skin, and adds to the pressure. In some cases blood will appear in the corn or callus as a brown–red stain (extravasation), and this is often an indication that an ulcer has developed or is about to develop under the hard skin.

Most foot ulcers will heal if a proper assessment is made to identify the under-lying cause of the ulcer (perhaps an ill-fitting shoe), and the cause removed. New, soft leather shoes might be used, or high plantar pressures offloaded with special insoles. Sometimes purpose-made footwear will be needed for deformed feet.

Common causes of foot injury

Accidental trauma may be difficult to avoid, but some injury can be pre-dicted and avoided. Those with neuropathy should take special care with hot water when taking a bath or shower, avoid toasting their feet in front of the fire or on heating pads or hot water bottles, and be especially careful to avoid sunburn.

The most common form of injury to the feet is that from ill-fitting foot-wear rubbing and causing hard skin or ulceration. Therefore, an assess-ment of footwear is essential. Shoes should be foot-shaped, deep and wide enough to accommodate any deformity, with no seams or internal stitches that can rub. Corns and calluses develop over a period of time, while a blister often will develop quickly in response to pressure in the form of fric-tion (shearing stress), which most have seen (one hopes in others only!) in response to trauma from a new pair of shoes worn to a wedding for the first time, for example.

Treatments

Nerve damage

There is no treatment available for peripheral neuropathy other than prevention by good diabetic control. Most studies show that good control of blood pressure, blood glucose, and reduction in cholesterol will help prevent the development of arterial disease, and contribute to reduction of nerve damage.

Painful neuropathy may be treated with medication such as amitriptyline, carbamazepine, gabapentin, topical capsaicin found in red chilli peppers, transcutaneous electrical nerve stimulation (TENS), electrical spinal cord stimulation or cognitive therapy.

Poor circulation

Stopping smoking will be the single most important step that a patient may undertake to help with prevention of arterial disease. Anti-platelet agents such as aspirin may be prescribed in suitable individuals to help reduce the clotting ability of some cells in the bloodstream. Surgical reconstruction is possible in some cases of arterial disease, and careful assessment should be undertaken earlier rather than later.

Peripheral angioplasty or percutaneous translumnial angioplasty (PTA) is a procedure that dilates or opens up a stenosis or narrowed/blocked artery by threading a thin tube (balloon catheter), after making an incision, into an

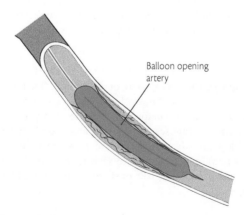

Balloon opening artery

Figure 6.6 Balloon angioplasty.

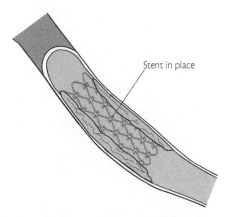

Stent in place

Figure 6.7 A stent.

artery in the leg and inflating it at the stenosis, or blocked area. The balloon pushes the plaque in the artery against the artery wall, widening the vessel. Sometimes a small mesh-like tube (stent) may be left in the artery to keep it open.

Another procedure that shaves plaque from inside the artery may also be used (endarterectomy). Sometimes the stenosis or block may be extensive, and bypass surgey will be necessary. Bypass surgery consists of the surgeon connecting artificial or transplanted vein and producing a detour around the blocked or stenosed artery. The blood then flows through this new vessel.

Often in diabetes it is the small blood vessels between the knee and ankle (distal) that become diseased, making surgery more difficult as the vessels become smaller as they travel to the foot. A bypass from the thigh to the foot is referred to as a distal bypass. Vascular surgery is not always successful, and a surgeon will advise the best course of action and type of surgery, and the risks involved.

Corns and calluses

Deformity and the pressure over time cause the thickening of the skin and, although regular podiatry is essential, simply removing the hard skin will not resolve the situation. The pressure will need to be reduced to prevent recurrence. The use of corn cures which contain acids is to be avoided as they burn into the skin and cause ulceration.

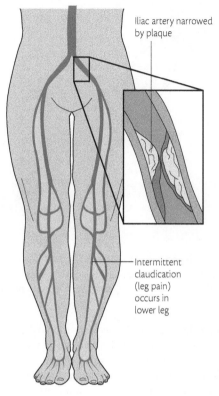

Iliac artery narrowed by plaque

Intermittent claudication (leg pain) occurs in lower leg

Figure 6.8 Peripheral arterial disease/stenosis.

Deformity and high pressure areas

It may be that special insoles are required to reduce pressure over the sole of the foot. Deep and wide shoes may be needed to accommodate any toe deformity, and specialist made-to-measure footwear may be needed to accommodate insoles.

Foot ulceration

Most foot ulcers will heal if a proper assessment is made to remove the underlying cause of the ulcer. Shoes need to be carefully chosen, and sometimes purpose-made footwear will be needed for deformed feet. It is a sad fact that people with sensory neuropathy continue to traumatize their feet and prevent

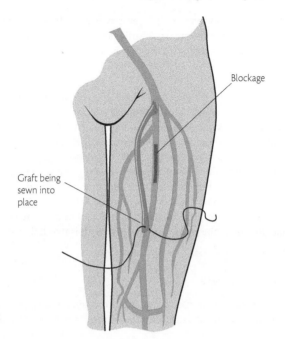

Figure 6.9 Bypass of a blocked artery.

them from healing because they cannot feel pain. The importance of resting and offloading the area cannot be overemphasized.

An ulcer may need to have any overlying hard skin or dead tissue removed (debridement), and the whole area should be cleaned and covered with a suitable dressing. It may be necessary for plaster casts, off-the-shelf replaceable plastic casts (air cast walkers), orthopaedic footwear and orthoses (insoles), healing shoes/sandals (Darco), or offloading felt padding to be used to offload pressure from ulcer sites to allow them to heal.

Those with foot ulcers failing to heal because of poor circulation need to be referred to a vascular surgeon to improve the circulation in order for the ulcer to heal.

Infection

Superficial foot infections need to be treated with oral antibiotics. If the infection is deep or flaring, then intravenous antibiotics will be needed, initially in hospital. Sometimes surgery will be necessary to drain pus or remove infected tissue and bone. A toe or part of the foot may need to be sacrificed to ensure healing. So time is of the essence: the earlier an infection is found and treated, the less chance serious surgery will be required.

Amputation

Amputation needs to be avoided if at all possible, but in some cases it may be the only way to avoid many months of misery. In some cases it is life-saving, because having infected tissues will cause general (systemic) illness. Amputation may be of the toe, foot, or lower leg, depending upon the spread of any infection and the blood supply. If the circulation is poor, it may be necessary to amputate to the nearest adequate blood vessels—this is why sometimes there is a need to remove the lower part of the leg altogether. However, even amputation should not be seen as a disaster. Artificial limbs, walking aids, and careful physiotherapy can lead to a restoration of near-normal life patterns. The younger and fitter the person, the more likely it is that full mobility will be restored.

Preventative foot care

Those with peripheral neuropathy cannot rely on pain sensation to register that something may be going awry. Alternative strategies need to be put in place.

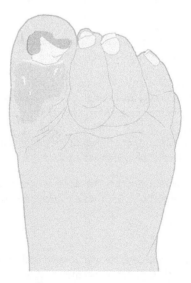

Figure 6.10 Ingrowing toe nail.

Walking barefoot, or in open sandals should be avoided. Every day someone needs to check that all is well—are there any signs of blisters, corns, calluses, cracks in the skin, or infection? Sometimes those with diabetes can manage this for themselves, but often there will be difficulties—poor eyesight or stiff limbs may mean that this task is a challenge. A mirror may help, but the image will appear far away. Someone else may need to take on this vital task. Any new suspicious changes detected in the feet should be referred to a nurse, podiatrist, or doctor.

Self-treatment with corn cures or razor blades should be avoided. Ingrowing toe nails are often caused by individuals cutting down the sides of the nail and leaving a spike behind. This then penetrates the tissue as the nail grows forward and the toe often becomes infected. Toe nails should be cut straight across and not too short.

> ## ❌ Myth
>
> **Cutting a V in the nail will resolve an ingrowing nail.**
>
> This is false. Those with ingrowing nails should consult a podiatrist.

Emollient creams can be used at least once a day on dry skin, particularly around the heels. Avoid using such creams between the toes, which should be kept dry.

In order to avoid trauma or injury, shoes should fit without any likelihood of rubbing or of constriction. It is good practice to check the inside of shoes for foreign objects or worn linings on a daily basis.

Holiday footcare advice

Some simple advice can prevent holidays being ruined by avoidable foot problems, most of which are caused by trauma or sunburn. A high factor sun cream is important, and care should be taken to avoid burning on hot surfaces such as sand or concrete. Walking around barefoot is crazy.

An emollient cream to prevent the skin drying out and cracking (see above) is a good plan, and new footwear that has not been worn before is dangerous. It is better to wear footwear that fits, than use new shoes that damage the feet. Special shoes will have been prescribed to reduce pressure and to prevent ulceration. That risk does not diminish just because one is not at home! Neuropathic feet may need special care—long walks and unaccustomed standing may wreck them in a very short time. They will need inspecting every day for signs of damage: cuts, discharge, changes in colour, redness, or swelling.

A first-aid kit containing an antiseptic, some sterile dressings, and tape is worth having close by. Medical help should be sought promptly—waiting to return home may spell disaster. Time is of the essence.

Conclusion

Careful foot care is mandatory in diabetes. If there is trauma to the feet, or if high pressure areas lead to ulceration, or if there is any trace of infection, then prompt treatment should prevent more serious consequences.

It is important that a health provider assesses the risk of foot problems at least once a year. There should be a screen for peripheral vascular disease, peripheral neuropathy, level of deformity, and advice about foot care and prevention of complications.

Eyes—retinopathy

Key points

- Tissue at the back of the eye called the retina has a rich blood supply and enables us to form images.

- The macula is a specialized part of the retina that produces the central focused part of any image.

- Diabetes may affect small vessels including those in the retina.

- There are various types of retinopathy found in diabetes, with some stages involving temporary reversible changes.

- Cataracts may also form in the lens at the front of the eye, obscuring vision over a long period of time.

- Improving blood glycaemic control reduces the risk of retinopathy.

- Regular eye examination is crucial to diagnosing and treating retinopathy before any complications or sight reduction.

What is retinopathy?

Diabetic retinopathy describes a collection of changes in the small vessels at the back of the eye (the retina) caused by diabetes, high blood pressure, or both. These changes are estimated to affect about 30% of the diabetic population, but usually have no effects on eyesight. However, serious problems can occur (estimated to be 2% in the UK diabetic population) which will need specialist treatment.

What causes retinopathy?

High levels of blood glucose found in diabetes can result in narrowing or blockage of the vessels at the back of the eye. The body's natural response is to produce new vessels—just as it would after any injury. But these new vessels can be delicate, tortuous, come forward into the eye, and are prone to leak. Bleeding from new fragile vessels into the jelly-like fluid (vitreous humour) in the middle of the eyeball may result in complete loss of vision in the worst affected cases—this is called 'vitreous haemorrhage'.

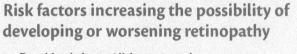

Risk factors increasing the possibility of developing or worsening retinopathy

◆ Poor blood glucose/diabetes control.

◆ Longer duration of diabetes.

◆ High blood pressure.

◆ Pregnancy.

◆ Alcohol.

◆ Recent cataract surgery.

Diabetic retinopathy

Retinopathy affecting the peripheral parts of the retina may be completely without symptoms until a newly formed vessel ruptures—at which point treatment becomes more complicated and less likely to be successful. This makes it important to look for signs of retinopathy on a regular basis in annual monitoring to diagnose and treat as early as possible. There are national schemes to ensure that this is carried out using digital photography, and the photographs are examined using trained graders.

Retinopathy can be divided into an early reversible 'background' stage which just requires repeat monitoring, and then more developed stages where treatment is indicated.

Type	Description	Common medical terms
Background retinopathy which may be reversible. Needs repeat monitoring	Blowing out of small areas in the walls of the tiny blood vessels	Microaneurysms or 'dots'
Established retinopathy. Needs referral and treatment in specialist centres	Small leaks of fluid from damaged blood vessels	Exudates
	Small bleeds from leaking vessels	Blot haemorrhages
	Some vessels may become blocked and prevent oxygen supply to parts of the retina	Cotton wool spots
	New vessels may form in areas of poor blood supply	Neovascularization
	New vessel formation at the front of the eye may alter fluid drainage from inside the eye	Diabetes-related glaucoma
	Large bleed into the eye causing sudden loss of vision	Vitreous haemorrhage

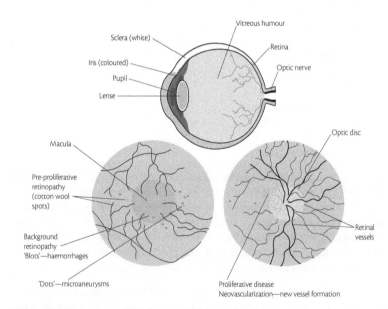

Figure 6.11 Eye anatomy with features of retinopathy.

How is retinopathy diagnosed and monitored?

The recommended annual eye check is usually carried out by an optician and involves two parts. First the visual 'acuity', or clarity of sight, is assessed using a selection of different lenses to correct any abnormality.

Secondly the retina is examined, either using a bright light source (ophthalmoscope) to examine directly, or using a retinal camera to record the view, presented as circular photographs, one of each eye. Either of these processes may involve using drops into the eye to open up the pupil and allow a better view. The photographs need to be sent off for grading, although an experienced optician can decide whether there are any major abnormalities.

How is retinopathy treated?

Blood pressure lowering and good glucose control are the first necessities in treating retinopathy. For established new vessels, laser treatment is indicated, and this is undertaken at specialist centres. The principles behind laser treatment are easy to understand—partly damaged tissues cause the body to react by producing new vessels, but scar tissue does not. In the same way, while a new cut on the arm is red and surrounded by new vessels, a scar is not. So laser therapy burns tiny scars on the back of the eye. These burns need to be away from the centre of vision, but they are very small and many hundreds can be delivered to an eye. Remarkably, although night vision may be affected, generally these burns do not impair vision in any noticeable way.

Vitreous haemorrhages cause sudden loss of vision because there is blood in the eye. This may sometimes be treated with bed rest, because part of the haemorrhage will clear naturally. However, in cases of persistent loss of vision, the vitreous can be removed entirely with specialist surgery. Early advice should always be sought after such visual loss.

Detached retina

With retinopathy the retina itself may tear away from the back of the eye. This can result in visual loss, especially of some particular part of the visual field. The retina can be re-attached with surgery or with laser treatment, so early referral to experts is manadatory.

Maculopathy

The macula is an important specialized part of the retina, almost in the middle, where vision is focused and the clear central part of an image is formed. This can also be affected by diabetes in a process called 'maculopathy', which may be seen as small bleeds (haemorrhages) or exudates (fluid leakages) in the macular area, or may just present with deterioration in vision but no obvious abnormality on direct view examination. In this last case, more complicated investigations may be needed to assess the extent of vessel damage. Maculopathy is complicated to treat, and needs referral to specialist centres.

Cataracts

Cataracts are caused by a clouding of the lens at the front of the eye. They are not found just in those with diabetes—they also occur with advancing age and in those who have been exposed to high levels of, usually tropical, sunlight. The clouding is often in the middle of the lens (cortical cataracts), so vision is affected and becomes quite misty. Because this mistiness is in the centre of the lens, those with these cataracts sometimes find that they can see better, paradoxically, in dim light. That is because the pupil of the eye is then bigger, and so the vision can be focused by the parts of the lens without the cataract.

Spoke cataracts, on the other hand, are quite different. These, as the name suggests, are like spokes of a wheel without a central hub. They may be detected when the eyes are examined—especially if the pupils are dilated. But they very rarely cause any visual problems, and are completely covered up by the iris (the coloured part of the eye around the pupil) in bright light—which is what is advised in these cases.

Central cortical cataracts can be removed and replaced by an artificial lens during a short surgical procedure carried out under local anaesthetic. This provides an immediate improvement in vision. Spoke cataracts need no treatment.

Cloudy vision early after diagnosis

Some of those diagnosed with diabetes find that their vision suddenly becomes very poor, and are alarmed that this is diabetic retinopathy or cataracts. This is very unlikely. Retinopathy is rare in the first 5 years of diabetes—though, of course, that is not the same as the first 5 years from diagnosis, which may have been delayed. The usual cause of poor vision early in treatment is that the blood glucose is coming under control quickly. When this happens, the sugar-saturated lens absorbs more fluid in the same way that dried sugary fruits will absorb water. The lens then becomes cloudy for a few days up to a few weeks. When the body settles to a new, steadier state of near-normal sugar, this cloudiness will clear. Therefore, it is important not to rush off and get new glasses in these first few weeks—the new lenses will be the wrong ones!

Kidneys—nephropathy

> ## ➲ Key points
>
> ◆ The kidneys act as filters to remove waste products from the body while retaining important components of blood.
>
> ◆ Diabetes can affect small vessels within the kidneys to cause loss of protein in the urine and, in advanced cases, kidney failure.
>
> ◆ The earliest stages of kidney failure or renal failure (nephropathy) can be diagnosed by a simple urine test for protein.
>
> ◆ Maintaining tight glycaemic and blood pressure control reduces the incidence of nephropathy.
>
> ◆ Treatment in the earliest stages can slow or potentially reverse nephropathy.

What is nephropathy?

Nephropathy is the medical term for diabetic kidney (renal) disease, which can occur in both types of diabetes. In type 1 diabetes it can take many years to develop, and is rarely seen in the first 10 years after diagnosis.

The kidneys function to filter the watery components of the blood and then recapture the glucose, salts, and much of the fluid component. What is left is the urine, which passes down a single tube from each kidney to the bladder. If the kidneys begin to be affected by diabetes, the filtering system becomes less effective and protein leaks through into the urine. This is microalbuminuria, where very small amounts of albumin (the most plentiful protein) are detected by laboratory analysis. Microalbuminuria can be present for many years without there being any progress to more serious disease.

With progression of nephropathy there is an increased protein loss, which can be detected by the urine dipstick analysis that is a routine part of diabetes outpatient clinics and GP surgery review appointments. A positive dipstick test is often followed up by sending the urine sample to the laboratory for further quantification of protein or a check that there is no urinary infection.

Functions of the kidneys

- Filtering the blood to rid it of waste products.

- Controlling blood pressure and blood volume.

- Producing hormone messages (erythropoietin) which go to the bone marrow to stimulate red blood cell production—without adequate levels of this hormone a person may become anaemic.

- Controlling bone health through vitamin D.

It is relatively common to discover small amounts of microalbuminuria in those with diabetes. If this progresses, as it does in some, there may be a requirement for dialysis or treatment by kidney transplantation. To reduce the risk of nephropathy developing, it is essential to maintain the overall health of the kidneys and the blood vessels supplying these organs. This includes general cardiovascular risk reduction (see page 128), in particular careful control of blood pressure. The kidneys are delicate and complicated organs, receiving between 20 and 25% of the total blood output from the heart.

There is a strong connection between the incidence of nephropathy and retinopathy (eye) complications, and a careful ophthalmic examination is essential when microalbuminuria is diagnosed.

How is nephropathy diagnosed?

- Nephropathy is diagnosed by detecting microalbuminuria in samples sent to a laboratory.

- More advanced nephropathy is found by detecting protein in the urine by dipsticks (proteinuria).

- A decline in kidney function results in an elevation of blood creatinine.

- Urea and blood potassium may be raised late in renal failure.

Symptoms of nephropathy

- Tiredness (often because of anaemia).

- Nausea and loss of appetite.

- Itchy skin.

- Swelling of ankles, hands, and eyelids owing to fluid build up.

What treatments are available?

- Blood pressure control becomes even more important when microalbuminuria is diagnosed. The force at which blood enters the kidneys can overstress the filtration system. It is advisable to keep the blood pressure below about 130/80 mmHg, and home measurements of blood pressure can provide useful information to assess the degree of effectiveness of various treatments. Home blood pressure machines can be bought relatively cheaply from chemists' stores, providing useful information for patient and doctor alike.

- The most common medications used to control blood pressure and slow the progression of diabetic nephropathy are ACE inhibitors. These act to reduce blood pressure, but can also have a protective effect on the kidneys before any elevation in blood pressure being seen.

- Careful control of blood glucose and lipids is important to reduce nephropathy and its progress.

- Hormonal changes occurring in the later stages of nephropathy can be counteracted by activated vitamin D for bone health.

- Injections of erythropoietin for red blood-cell production, as required. Regular monitoring while on these therapies is important to prevent over- or undertreatment.

What is dialysis?

If kidney function deteriorates further, it may be necessary to filter waste products artificially. This process is known as dialysis. There are two forms of this: peritoneal dialysis and haemodialysis.

- Peritoneal dialysis uses large volumes of warmed fluid inserted into the abdominal cavity by a specially sited tube. Waste products from the blood, including compounds called urea and creatinine, enter this fluid, which is then drained off. This procedure requires a careful routine performed up to four times per day. Cleanliness around the tube site is essential to prevent infection. Peritoneal dialysis does allow independence to be maintained—it can be easily carried out at home after some training.

◆ Haemodialysis is a far more effective way of removing waste products from the blood, as it works by filtering the blood through a complicated machine. However, this takes up to 8 hours on each occasion and needs to be repeated on average three times a week. Initially this process requires a small operation to join a vein and artery in an accessible position, often the forearm, to allow the dialysis machine to be attached. Then the person is restricted to the hospital bed for the length of the filtration.

Renal (kidney) transplantation

Dialysis is time-consuming and expensive. It is better if a new kidney can be transplanted because this allows a near normal lifestyle. Kidneys need to be donated, however, and there is currently a shortage of donors. When a kidney does become available—often after road traffic accidents—the tissue needs to be matched as well as possible to the person receiving the transplantation. As a result kidneys can be moved large distances around the country to make sure that the match is as good as possible. Those waiting for a kidney have their names on a waiting list—and this list is used to get the best match. So some people can wait on the list for a long time, while others may, by chance, get a good match in a short time.

After transplantation, careful monitoring is needed. Blood pressure and blood glucose need to be controlled so that the new kidney does not get diabetic disease and, even with relatively good matches, some form of immunosuppression will be needed. This involves taking additional tablets.

Erectile dysfunction and female sexual dysfunction

➲ Key points

◆ Erectile dysfunction is relatively common in the general population but more so in men with diabetes.

◆ Female sexual dysfunction is under-recognized but is known to occur in a significant proportion of the female diabetic population.

◆ Diabetes may affect blood vessel and nerve function required for arousal and orgasm in both sexes.

Potential causes of sexual dysfunction affecting men or women include:

- Physical—surgery or injury to the genital, pelvic or spine regions, infection or inflammation of local structures.

- Hormonal—hormonal deficiencies.

- Lifestyle—smoking, alcohol, recreational drugs.

- Medication—treatment for heart disease, control of blood pressure, anti-depressants, sedatives, tranquillizers.

- Psychological—tiredness, stress, anxiety, depression, relationship difficulties often with secondary feelings of guilt, inadequacy, or embarrassment.

There are several forms of effective treatment available:

- Lifestyle changes—adequate exercise, relaxation, reduced stress, improved relationship communication, reduced alcohol excess, stopping smoking.

- For erectile dysfunction—tablets, injections, hormonal pellets, or surgical implants, depending on the individual cause and situation.

- Vacuum devices available for both sexes.

- Relaxation and stress management techniques may be useful.

- Counselling can address emotional issues surrounding such a diagnosis and the effects of this on one or both partners in the relationship.

> I suppose one of the problems is the sexual side of diabetes, in that this does have a great effect on your relationship—and diabetes unfortunately can affect these aspects of your life. But there is help available if you only just know where to go and where to ask for it.
>
> Anon

What is erectile dysfunction?

Erectile dysfunction (ED) is an inability to achieve and/or maintain an erection suitable for sexual intercourse. ED and female sexual dysfunction (FSD) are more common in people with diabetes. This section explores the possible causes, treatments available, and emotional issues that may be involved.

Diabetes can affect the small nerves to the sexual organs, with the result that erections and sexual sensations are impaired. ED may often be the result of diabetes alone, but is important to consider other causes. There will need to be an individual assessment including medical history, physical examination, and blood tests.

ED is the most common sexual problem facing about 1 in 10 men in the UK at any one time and affecting almost 50% of men at some point in their lives. ED can have many different causes, including tiredness, stress, various medications, hormonal problems, and blood vessel disease. It also becomes more common with age, when arousal tends to take longer anyway, with reduced blood flow producing a less firm erection. In many cases there is a decreasing testosterone level. Although many couples find that discussing the subject of sexual activity is difficult, it is important to mention it to health professionals as ED can have profound effects on relationships, and several effective treatment options can be made available if it is identified as an issue.

What causes ED?

Physical causes

The physical process of erection relies on increased blood flow into, with temporarily reduced blood flow out of, the penis. Any damage to the blood vessels supplying this organ may result in ED. Diabetes can cause narrowing of the vessels. The process of arousal also relies on intact sensation provided by local nerve supply. The nerves can be damaged by poor blood supply when the small vessels supplying the nerves are affected by diabetes. Smoking causes accelerated narrowing of the vessels, and can adversely affect sexual arousal, so stopping is important.

Hormonal causes

A low testosterone level may be the cause of ED in some men, especially after some surgical procedures, trauma to the testes, bladder, pelvis, prostate gland, or spine, prolonged ill health, or increasing age. Testosterone is the major male hormone defining characteristic sexual development, muscle size and strength, voice deepening, and hair distribution. This hormone is produced in the testes (testicles) of a man, and the production increases during puberty to bring about the changes characteristically associated with adult development. Testosterone levels peak in early adulthood, slowly reducing into older age. Testosterone is produced in larger amounts in the early morning, with a gradual reduction expected during the day.

Thyroid or pituitary gland abnormalities can also result in reduced testosterone production, so tests should be undertaken to check that these are normal.

Lifestyle causes

A lack of exercise, excessive weight gain, smoking, the use of some recreational drugs, or excessive alcohol intake can reduce desires and cause ED. Stress at work or home, depression in any form, or tiredness including physical over-activity can contribute to any potential physical impairment, making the problem worse. Sexual activity needs time and relaxation. It is worth considering whether this has been prioritized, and if not, taking steps to find the best time and environment.

Medication

Sexual desire may be directly reduced as a side effect of some medications, particularly those used to treat heart disease and to reduce blood pressure. Antidepressants, sedatives, or tranquillizers can all have an adverse effect. A doctor should review the list of medications if there is a problem with ED.

Psychological causes

Feelings of tiredness, stress, or frank depression all have an impact on sexual desire and can have profound effects on relationships including loss of interest in sex or in a sexual partner. These situations may then be further complicated by personal feelings of guilt, inadequacy, or embarrassment. The emotional difficulties associated with the diagnosis, treatment, or management of diabetes may result in altered body image, or reduced self-confidence may affect relationship harmony. Intervention should be a priority.

Treatment options for ED

These can best be fully discussed with a doctor or nurse with a specialist interest in diabetes or ED. However, it can be a difficult subject to discuss, and starting with a local GP may be the preferred option. A medical history and examination begin the process to identify possible causes of ED. Blood tests may follow to measure testosterone and other hormonal factors as well as indicators of glucose control. Many of the issues involved in causing ED can be improved by simple measures such as:

* Improving lifestyle:
  * Adequate physical activity
  * Relaxation

- ◆ Reducing alcohol intake
- ◆ Stopping smoking

◆ Improving communication with partner.

◆ Complementary counselling or therapy.

Medical therapy

This is aimed at increasing blood flow to and reducing blood flow from the penis on a temporary and reversible basis. Tablets such as Viagra and Cialis can be very effective.

> For me, Viagra has done a great deal of good. It's enabled me to play a full part. My performance is also a great deal better than it was.
>
> Anon

Alternative treatments include vacuum devices, injection into the shaft or ure-thral application (into the tube in the centre of the penis, such as Muse), or medication to produce a similar effect. In testosterone deficiency, replacement of the hormone is the treatment, in injection, implant, patch, or gel forms.

What is female sexual dysfunction?

Although far less well recognized, FSD may affect up to a quarter of the female diabetic population, producing pain on intercourse or altering any aspect of desire, arousal, or orgasm. Although women with diabetes are con-sidered to be affected twice as often by some or all of these issues than those women without diabetes, many of the causes may be similar and easily addressed. Discussion of these issues with a doctor or healthcare professional can feel embarrassing, but can be very worthwhile, and the choice of a female doctor for the consultation may reduce this initial awkwardness. As with male ED, a holistic view of the person is essential to effective treatment of FSD.

What causes FSD?

Physical causes

Local causes include gynaecological inflammation, infection, surgery, or injury. Urinary tract infections or vaginal thrush infection may cause pain and dis-comfort with sex, and will need treatment. Thrush treatment will need to be given to both partners if a recurrence of infection is to be avoided. Any recent trauma of giving birth may affect attitudes to sex, and care will be needed from partners.

Hormonal causes

Vaginal dryness may cause painful intercourse, and may reflect a low oestrogen level, which may be helped by hormone replacement therapy. Low oestrogen may also affect sexual desire and self-image. Local creams containing oestrogen are also available, but it is important to judge carefully about oestrogen therapy, as other risks may increase.

Other causes

These are similar to those for male ED, and include medications, psychological causes, lack of exercise, weight gain, smoking, the use of some recreational drugs, or excessive alcohol. As with ED, stress at work or home, depression in any form, and tiredness including physical overactivity may all contribute. It is, as with ED, worth making sure that time and opportunity are prioritized in order to overcome stress elements.

What treatments are available for FSD?

◆ Psychosexual counselling and relaxation techniques can be very effective if the issues are primarily stress-related or if secondary feelings of inadequacy exist.

◆ Lifestyle management including improving physical activity, diet, any weight issues—excessive weight or underweight—stopping smoking, and reducing alcohol intake if this is excessive.

◆ Review of current medication to reduce possible effects on sexual function.

At present there are no medications used in the treatment of FSD, although oestrogen replacement in oral, patch, or cream form may be indicated. Vacuum devices do exist to encourage increased blood flow.

7

What care to expect

In the UK, the National Health Service aims to give equal treatment to all regardless of age, gender, ethnicity, religious beliefs, disability, or sexuality. This applies to people with diabetes, although some inequality does still exist.

> **❓ FAQ**
>
> ## Who will provide my diabetes care? Will I have to go to hospital?
>
> In the UK, the health service is divided into Primary Care (your local GP or health centre) and Secondary Care (hospital- or specialist-based). Much of your routine diabetes care may be provided by your local GP. Different people may need different levels of care, and the broad categories are shown below:
>
> Primary care: Most people with newly diagnosed type 2 diabetes
>
> People with type 2 diabetes that is stable
>
> People with type 1 diabetes who choose to see their GP
>
> Secondary care: Most people with type 1 diabetes
>
> Pregnant women and women with gestational diabetes
>
> People with type 2 diabetes needing specialist input
>
> Local areas may have different guidelines, and your local Primary Care Trust (PCT) should be able to supply further information.

Will I see my own GP?

In many health centres there is a specific GP and Practice Nurse with a specialist interest in diabetes, and they usually run diabetes clinics. You may not see your own doctor, but you will see a health professional with experience in diabetes.

Who will I see if I have to go to hospital?

Many hospitals now have diabetes clinics, and these include a team of health professionals who specialize in the management of different aspects of diabetes. Members of the team can include:

* Consultant or specialist doctors

* Diabetes specialist nurses (DSNs)

* Dietitian

* Ophthamologist/optometrist

* Podiatrist/chiropodist

* Psychologist/behavioural therapist

Remember—you are the most important member of the diabetes team!

You may not need to see all members of the diabetes team at each hospital visit, but you will usually see a doctor and they can refer you to other specialities if necessary.

What care to expect at diagnosis

People with type 1 diabetes will usually be referred to a specialist hospital clinic. They should receive a full medical examination and education from a DSN and a dietitian. The initial consultation should include:

* Medical history and examination.

* Prescription for insulin, insulin pen, or syringe.

* Blood glucose meter (in some centres these are supplied free of charge and in others people are expected to purchase their own) and prescription of blood-testing strips.

◆ Education about injection technique, and frequency and amount of insulin injections.

◆ Education about use of the meter to measure blood glucose.

◆ Explanation of the causes, symptoms, and treatment of hypoglycaemia.

◆ Lifestyle information, especially dietary factors.

◆ Information about driving, employment, and insurance.

◆ Some assessment of impact on quality of life and recognition of any psychosocial issues.

People with type 2 diabetes seen in primary care can expect a consultation with a GP and a practice nurse, and this should include:

◆ Medical history and examination.

◆ Prescription for suitable medication (if necessary).

◆ Blood glucose meter (if appropriate—see Chapter 4).

◆ Education on medication including doses, frequency, and any side effects.

◆ Explanation of the causes, symptoms, and treatment of hypoglycaemia if relevant.

◆ Lifestyle information including diet, physical activity, and weight loss.

◆ Some assessment of impact on quality of life and recognition of any psychosocial issues.

What care to expect during routine clinic appointments

Routine follow-up appointments are usually arranged according to individual need; those with stable control may find that they receive an annual review and others may need to attend more regularly. Routine appointments will usually involve a review of medical treatment, offer support, and a chance to discuss any lifestyle factors, and may include some blood tests for A1c, lipid levels, and any other relevant factors.

Annual review

Everyone with diabetes should be offered an annual review. This consultation should include biochemical tests, physical assessments, and ongoing education.

Biochemical (blood and urine) tests

◆ A1c to measure long-term blood glucose control.

◆ Urine and blood tests to assess kidney function.

◆ Blood test to measure lipid levels (total cholesterol, HDL cholesterol, and triglycerides) and assess risk of heart disease.

Physical examinations

◆ Body weight is measured and usually reported both in kilograms and as BMI.

◆ Blood pressure should be taken to assess risk of cardiovascular disease.

◆ Legs and feet are examined to assess skin, blood, and nerve supply.

◆ Eyes should be examined regularly by means of a retinal photograph. In the UK, there is now a system in place to ensure that all people with diabetes should have a retinal photograph taken annually.

◆ People who take insulin should have their injection sites examined.

Changes in the above assessments can be evaluated and may need referral to a specialist. Any issues with kidney function may require a referral to a renal unit. Raised blood lipid levels and blood pressure may require medication to reduce the risk of cardiovascular disease, problems with the legs and feet may require the services of a podiatrist, and changes in eye photographs may result in referral to a specialist eye unit.

Ongoing education and well-being

The following factors should also be included in the annual review:

◆ Current medication and any necessary adjustment.

◆ Management of diabetes including self-monitoring and hypoglycaemia.

◆ General well-being and any outstanding issues including smoking, weight management, diet, alcohol, physical activity, and sexual problems.

❓ FAQ

What kind of education and support should I expect now I have diabetes?

In the UK, the Department of Health recommends that all people with diabetes should receive structured education. Provision of education is usually available at a local level. People with type 1 diabetes may be invited to a DAFNE course (Does Adjustment for Normal Eating), or to a local education programme. Education programmes for people with type 1 diabetes usually cover carbohydrate counting and insulin adjustment, and management of exercise, illness, and hypoglycaemia. People with type 2 diabetes should have structured education offered at diagnosis, often through the DESMOND (Diabetes Education and Self-Management for Ongoing and Newly Diagnosed) or the X-PERT programmes. Both these programmes are nationally recognized in the UK, although there may be a different programme offered in your local area. The programmes for type 2 diabetes usually include topics such as explaining diabetes, medication, diet and physical activity, and also address quality of life. You can ask your GP, practice nurse, or hospital clinic about local initiatives.

8

The future

The future for someone with diabetes is much brighter today than it ever was before. The therapeutic advances mean that we now understand the crucial need for ongoing care in diabetes. Glucose control is much easier with modern therapies, and the use of agents to keep blood pressure and blood fats under control means that the long-term risks of diabetes are reducing year on year. The dangers of smoking (with or without diabetes) have become much more apparent in recent years, with the realization that continuing smokers have a 1 in 2 chance of dying of smoking-related disease; so there is a concerted campaign on that front as well.

All this shows that the outlook is rosier than it ever was. However, the real questions about a cure remain unanswered. In type 1 diabetes, although we know a huge amount about how autoimmunity works—essentially how the body makes a mistake over what is self and what is not—we still do not know enough about how to stop the process of destruction of the beta-cells. Similarly, in type 2 diabetes, we know that the beta-cells are not working hard enough to produce the insulin we need, yet we have only a few clues about the processes involved in their progressive failure.

Where will the research lead us? In type 1 diabetes there is a big research effort in trying to establish mechanisms of onset and techniques for prevention. Immune systems can be tricked in several ways—immunization works on the basis of pre-exposure to a small quantity of a disease protein from, for example, mumps or measles, so that the first time the body comes across the disease for real the viruses are wiped out very fast. Type 1 diabetes presents the opposite problem! We need to train the body that beta-cells are not to be wiped out. We know that mechanism exists because it is the basis of all immune selectivity. Can we re-programme the body so that it does not make a mistake? That is quite a challenge.

Could we replace the beta-cells? Islet transplantation shows us that this is not only possible but that those who have had the procedure benefit from better glucose control. Nevertheless, we do not have enough islets to transplant except in a very few cases, and we desperately need to solve the problem that we have to use immunosuppression in the long term to prevent rejection of the new tissue. Islet transplantation is now available for a few people, and is directed at those who have recurrent intractable, disabling hypoglycaemia. It is only available to such people at the moment because of a shortage of human islets (obtained from organ donors), and because immunosuppression means that there are risks as well as benefits.

Could we build new beta-cells? Again, it seems possible from stem-cell knowledge that we could, and that it might even be possible to alter the surface proteins of the cells so that the immune system would not recognize them as 'foreign'. However, the work so far has been disappointingly slow. Even when cells that can make insulin have been found, they produce about 1000 times less insulin than the normal beta-cell. It also seems that we need islets rather than beta-cells for good functional capacity, and so we would need to undertake biological engineering for several different cell types.

In type 2 diabetes there has been a surge of activity relating to new ways of stimulating the beta-cells, the most hopeful to date being those agents that mimic the naturally occurring gut hormone, GLP-1. GLP-1 seems to sensitize the beta-cell to glucose so that more insulin is produced during high glucose exposure, but interestingly the amplification decreases as the glucose gets near to normal. In some test-tube experiments, GLP-1 seems to improve the survivability of the cells, so this would be a particularly efficacious treatment were this to be true in clinical practice. Whether this happens remains a matter of some contention and therefore of strong ongoing research activity.

New types of medications for type 2 diabetes

Exenatide (Byetta) is the first of a new class of medications available that mimic the effects of incretins. Incretins are hormones that are produced by the intestine and released into the blood in response to food. An example of an incretin is human glucagon-like peptide-1 (GLP-1). GLP-1 reduces glucose levels in the blood by four mechanisms:

Increases insulin secretion from pancreas.

Slows absorption of glucose from intestine.

Reduces action of glucagon (glucagon is a hormone that increases glucose production by the liver).

Reduces appetite and may help weight loss.

Exenatide is a synthetic hormone that acts like GLP-1. It can be used to improve glycaemic control when a person is on maximum oral medications. It is given by a twice daily injection under the skin, initially at a dose of 5 mcg, which can be increased to 10 mcg after a month. It is given an hour before breakfast or dinner and can be injected into the thigh, abdomen, or upper arm. One advantage of this type of agent is that hypoglycaemia is very rare. Its effect on appetite may result in some weight loss.

As one of exenatide's actions is to slow the transit of food and other drugs through the intestine, it can interfere with the absorption of drugs that are taken orally. Therefore it is recommended that oral tablets are taken one hour before exenatide is given. The most common side effect is nausea (which tends to occur at higher doses and reduces over time). There have been reports of associated acute pancreatitis, so it is recommended that a doctor should be seen if a person on exenatide is suffering with severe persistent abdominal pain. It should not be used by pregnant or breast-feeding mothers.

Sitagliptin (Januvia) is the first of another new class of medications that works by a similar mechanism to exenatide. These oral drugs are called the DPP-4 inhibitors and work by blocking the action of the enzyme dipeptidyl peptidase 4. This enzyme inactivates the hormone discussed above, GLP-1, so that in principle it has all the actions ascribed to exenatide but is weaker and has no effect on body weight. It can be taken with metformin alone, or a glitazone alone, and is given at a dose of 100 mg once daily. The main side effect is nausea, which may be more pronounced when given in combination with metformin. Flatulence and fluid retention have also been reported.

Exenatide and sitagliptin offer new strategies for treating diabetes and increasing numbers of patients are using them. NICE recommends exenatide as an alternative to insulin when maximum oral medications are not working. Sitagliptin can be thought of as an add-on therapy to metformin or a glitazone, when other more established oral combinations are still giving inadequate glycaemic control.

In the world of genetic research there are huge strides in understanding the 'blueprint' and the codes for health and disease. The research allows us to find ways of altering disease processes because it identifies new 'targets' for pharmaceutical agents. We may be able to modify the genetic codes in some individuals, but this is still some way off. Nevertheless, knowing the blueprint in any individual will allow us to assess risk and perhaps allow early or even pre-disease interventions.

Can we stop the epidemic of type 2 diabetes? It certainly seems likely that we could slow it significantly by changing our lifestyles away from the sedentary, and towards a more balanced, and less calorie-rich, eating pattern. The environment needs to be enhanced to help us achieve this: food labelling needs to be improved, facilities such as cycle lanes and parks need to be enhanced, families where diabetes is found in many generations may need special counselling, and early therapeutic interventions may help some at particular high risk. All these changes will require a shift of our priorities and a concerted investment by governments and by individuals.

What about healthcare for those with diabetes? Here there is a huge challenge. The World Health Organization estimates that there will be over 200 million people with type 2 diabetes by the year 2015. How will all these people be looked after and how will we be able to treat so many? Governments will need to be encouraged to provide services that are appropriate for all their population, and they will need to ensure that general practice care is integrated with specialist care. In a widening epidemic, there will be a temptation to reduce services to individuals and to aim for quantity of care rather than quality. We need to be aware that such trends are possible, and we need to become vocal advocates of high quality for all.

Appendix

Useful resources

Diabetes UK Central Office

Macleod House
10 Parkway
London NW1 7AA
Tel: 020 7424 1000
Fax: 020 7424 1001
E-mail: info@diabetes.org.uk
www.diabetes.org.uk

National Institute for Health and Clinical Excellence

Mid City Place
71 High Holborn
London WC1V 6NA
Tel: 020 7067 5800
E-mail: nice@nice.org.uk
www.nice.org.uk

NHS Direct

NHS Direct Line: 0845 4647
www.nhsdirect.nhs.uk

NHS 24 (Scotland)

Tel: 08454 242424
www.nhs24.com

International Diabetes Federation (IDF)

Avenue Emile De Mot 19

B-1000 Brussels

Belgium

Tel: +32-2-53855111

Fax: +32-2-5385114

www.idf.org

American Diabetes Association (ADA)

ATTN: National Call Center

1701 North Beauregard Street

Alexandria, VA 22311

USA

www.diabetes.org

The Diabetes Monitoring Forum

www.dmforum.org.uk

Driver and Vehicle Licensing Agency

DVLA

Swansea SA99 1TU

www.dvla.gov.uk

Driver and Vehicle Agency (Northern Ireland)

Driver Licensing Division

County Hall

Castlerock Road

Coleraine

Co. Londonderry BT51 3TB

Tel: 0845 402 4000

www.dvani.gov.uk

Foreign and Commonwealth Office

Travel advice at www.fco.gov.uk

Diabetes Research & Wellness Foundation

101–102 Northney Marina
Hayling Island
Hampshire PO11 0NH
Tel: 023 92 637 808
www.drwf.org.uk

Juvenile Diabetes Research Foundation

19 Angel Gate City Road
London EC1V 2PT
Tel: 020 7713 2030
Fax: 020 7713 2031
www.jdrf.org.uk

Insulin Dependent Diabetes Trust

PO Box 294
Northampton NN1 4XS
Tel: 01604 622837
www.iddtinternational.org

Diabetes Stories: an oral history website telling the stories of people living with diabetes

www.diabetes-stories.co.uk

Equality and Human Rights Commission (formally Disability Rights Commission)

www.equalityhumanrights.com

Equality and Human Rights Commission Disability Helpline (England)

Freepost MID02164

Stratford upon Avon CV37 9BR

Tel: 08457 622 633

Textphone: 08457 622 644

(Wales)

Equality and Human Rights Commission Helpline Wales

Freepost RRLR-UEYB-UYZL

1st Floor

3 Callaghan Square

Cardiff CF10 5BT

Tel: 0845 604 8810

Textphone: 0845 604 8820

(Scotland)

Equality and Human Rights Commission Helpline Scotland

Freepost RRLL-GYLB-UJTA

The Optima Building

58 Robertson Street

Glasgow G2 8DU

Tel: 0845 604 5510

Textphone: 0845 604 5520

Department of Health

www.dh.gov.uk

Royal National Institute of Blind People (RNIB)

105 Judd Street

London WC1H 9NE

Tel: 020 7388 1266

Fax: 020 7388 2034

www.rnib.org.uk

British Heart Foundation (BHF)

14 Fitzhardinge Street
London W1H 6DH
Tel: 020 7935 0185
www.bhf.org.uk

Kidney Research UK

Kings Chambers
Priestgate
Peterborough PE1 1FG
Tel: 0845 070 7601
www.kidneyresearchuk.org

The National Kidney Federation (NKF)

6 Stanley Street
Worksop
Notts S81 7HX
Tel: 01909 487795
Fax: 0845 601 02 09

Glossary

A1c A blood test that gives an indication of average blood glucose levels over 10–12 weeks.

ACE inhibitor A type of drug used to lower blood pressure. Studies indicate that it may also help prevent or slow the progression of kidney disease in people with diabetes.

Acetone A chemical formed in the blood when the body uses fat instead of glucose for energy. Acetone passes through the body into the urine. Someone with a lot of acetone in the body can have breath that smells fruity and is called 'acetone breath'. See also: Ketone bodies.

Acidosis Too much acid in the body. For a person with diabetes, this can lead to diabetic ketoacidosis (DKA). See also: Diabetic ketoacidosis.

Albuminuria More than normal amounts of a protein called albumin in the urine. Albuminuria may be a sign of kidney disease.

Alpha-cell A type of cell in the pancreas (in areas called the islets of Langerhans). Alpha-cells make and release a hormone called glucagon, which raises the level of glucose in the blood.

Angiopathy Disease of the blood vessels (arteries, veins, and capillaries) that occurs when someone has diabetes for a long time.

Antibodies Proteins that the body makes to protect itself from foreign substances.

Antigens Substances that cause an immune response in the body. The body 'sees' the antigens as harmful or foreign. To fight them, the body produces antibodies, which attack and try to eliminate the antigens.

Artery A large blood vessel that carries blood from the heart to other parts of the body.

Asymptomatic No symptoms; no clear sign of disease present.

Atherosclerosis One of many diseases in which fat builds up in the large and medium sized arteries. This build up of fat may slow down or stop blood flow.

Autoimmune disease Disorder of the body's immune system in which the immune system mistakenly attacks and destroys body tissue that it believes to be foreign.

Autonomic neuropathy A disease of the nerves affecting mostly the internal organs such as the bladder muscles, the cardiovascular system, the digestive tract, and the genital organs.

Background retinopathy Early stage of diabetic retinopathy; usually does not impair vision.

Basal rate Refers to a continuous supply of low levels of insulin, as in insulin pump therapy.

Beta-cell A type of cell in the pancreas in areas called the islets of Langerhans. Beta-cells make and release insulin, a hormone that controls the level of glucose in the blood.

Blood glucose Glucose is the major source of energy for living cells and is carried to each cell through the bloodstream. Glucose is largely derived from carbohydrate foods.

Blood glucose meter A machine that helps test how much glucose is in the blood.

Blood glucose monitoring A way of testing how much glucose is in the blood.

Body mass index (BMI) A measure used to evaluate body weight relative to a person's height. BMI is used to find out if a person is underweight, normal weight, overweight, or obese.

Blood vessels Tubes that act like a system of roads or canals to carry blood to and from all parts of the body. The three main types of blood vessel are arteries, veins, and capillaries. The heart pumps blood through these vessels so that the blood can carry with it oxygen and nutrients that the cells need, or take away waste that the cells do not need.

Bolus An extra amount of insulin taken to cover rises in blood glucose, such as those that occur after eating.

C-peptide A substance that the pancreas releases into the bloodstream in equal amounts to insulin. A test of C-peptide levels will show how much insulin the body is making.

Calcium channel blocker A drug used to lower blood pressure.

Calorie Energy that comes from food. Some foods have more calories than others. Fats have many calories, and most green leafy vegetables have few.

Carbohydrate One of the three main classes of foods and a source of energy. Carbohydrate foods are mainly sugars and starches that the body breaks down into glucose.

Carbohydrate counting A method of meal planning for people with diabetes based on counting the number of grams of carbohydrate in food.

Cardiologist A doctor who sees and takes care of people with heart disease; a heart specialist.

Cardiovascular Relating to the heart and blood vessels (arteries, veins, and capillaries); the circulatory system.

Carpal tunnel syndrome A nerve disorder affecting the hand that may occur in people with diabetes; caused by a pinched nerve.

Cataract Clouding of the lens of the eye.

Cerebrovascular disease Damage to the blood vessels in the brain, resulting in a stroke.

Charcot foot A foot complication associated with diabetic neuropathy that results in destruction of joints and soft tissue.

Cholesterol A fat-like substance found in blood, muscle, liver, brain, and other tissues in people and animals. The body makes and needs some cholesterol. Too much cholesterol, however, may cause fat to build up in the artery walls and result in a disease that slows or stops the flow of blood.

Coma An unconscious state. May be caused by a high or low level of glucose in the blood.

Contraindication A condition that makes a treatment not helpful or even harmful.

Creatinine A chemical found in the blood and passed in the urine. A test of the amount of creatinine in blood or in blood and urine may indicate kidney disease.

CSII: continuous subcutaneous insulin infusion See: Insulin pump.

Dawn phenomenon A sudden rise in blood glucose levels in the early morning hours.

Diabetes Control and Complications Trial (DCCT) A 10-year study (1983–1993) funded by the National Institute of Diabetes and Digestive and Kidney Diseases to assess the effects of intensive therapy on the long-term complications in those with type 1 diabetes. The study proved that intensive management of type 1 diabetes prevents or slows the development of eye, kidney and nerve damage caused by diabetes.

Diabetes mellitus A disease that occurs when the body is not able to utilize glucose for energy due to an absolute or relative lack of insulin.

Diabetic ketoacidosis (DKA) Severe, out-of-control diabetes caused by lack of insulin leading to high blood glucose levels.

Diabetogenic Causing diabetes; some drugs cause blood glucose to rise, resulting in diabetes.

Diabetologist A doctor who sees and treats people with diabetes mellitus.

Diagnosis The term used when a doctor finds that a person has a certain medical problem or disease.

Dialysis A method for removing waste such as urea from the blood when the kidneys can no longer do the job.

Dietitian An expert in nutrition who helps people plan the kinds and amounts of foods to eat. A state-registered dietitian (SRD) has special qualifications.

Diuretic A drug that increases the flow of urine to rid the body of extra fluid.

Endogenous Grown or made inside the body. Insulin made by a person's own pancreas is endogenous insulin.

Epidemiology The study of a disease that deals with patterns in the general population.

Euglycaemia A normal level of glucose in the blood.

Exogenous Grown or made outside the body; for instance, insulin that is made by manufacturers is exogenous insulin for people.

Fasting blood glucose test A method for finding out how much glucose is in the blood. The test is usually done in the morning before the person has eaten.

Fats One of the three main classes of food and a source of energy in the body. Fats help the body use some vitamins and keep the skin healthy. They also serve as energy stores for the body.

Fatty acids A basic unit of fats. When insulin levels are too low or there is not enough glucose to use for energy, the body burns fatty acids for energy.

Fibre A substance found in foods that come from plants. Fibre helps in the digestive process and is thought to lower cholesterol and help control blood glucose.

Foot care Taking special steps to avoid foot problems such as sores, cuts, bunions and calluses.

Fundus of the eye The back or deep part of the eye, including the retina.

Funduscopy A test to look at the back area of the eye to see if there is any damage to the vessels that bring blood to the retina. The doctor uses a device called an ophthalmoscope to check the eye.

Gangrene The death of body tissue caused by a loss of blood flow.

Gastroparesis A form of nerve damage that affects the stomach. Food is not digested properly and does not move through the stomach in a normal way, resulting in vomiting, nausea or bloating, and interfering with diabetes management. See also: Autonomic neuropathy.

Gene A basic unit of heredity.

Genetic Relating to genes.

Gestation The length of pregnancy.

Gestational diabetes mellitus (GDM) A type of diabetes mellitus that can occur when a woman is pregnant.

Glaucoma An eye disease associated with increased pressure within the eye. Glaucoma can damage the optic nerve and cause impaired vision and blindness.

Glomerular filtration rate Measure of the kidneys' ability to filter and remove waste products.

Glucagon A hormone that raises the level of glucose in the blood.

Glucose A simple sugar found in the blood. It is the body's main source of energy.

Glucose tolerance test A test to see if a person has diabetes.

Glycogen A substance made up of sugars. It is stored in the liver and muscles, and releases glucose into the blood when needed by cells.

Glycogenesis (or glucogenesis) The process by which glycogen is formed from glucose.

Glycosuria Having glucose in the urine.

Haemaglobin A1c (HbA1c) See A1c.

Haemodialysis A mechanical method of cleaning the blood for people who have kidney disease.

Home blood glucose monitoring A way a person can test how much glucose is in the blood. Also called self-monitoring of blood glucose.

Homeostatis When the body is working as it should because all of its systems are in balance.

Hormone A chemical released by special cells to tell other cells what to do. For instance, insulin is a hormone made by the beta-cells in the pancreas. When released, insulin tells other cells to use glucose for energy.

Human insulin Man-made insulins that are similar to insulin produced in the body.

Hyperglycaemia High levels of blood glucose.

Hyperlipidaemia Too high a level of fats (lipids) in the blood.

Hypertension Blood pressure that is above the normal range.

Hypoglycaemia Low levels of blood glucose.

Hypotension Low blood pressure or a sudden drop in blood pressure.

Impaired glucose tolerance (IGT) Blood glucose levels higher than normal but not high enough to be called diabetes.

Impotence Inability to achieve or maintain an erection.

Incidence How often a disease occurs; the number of new cases of a disease among a certain group of people for a certain period of time.

Insulin A hormone that helps the body use glucose for energy.

Insulin pen An insulin injection device the size of a pen that includes a needle and holds a vial of insulin. It can be used instead of syringes for giving insulin injections.

Insulin pump A device that delivers a continuous supply of insulin into the body.

Insulin resistance The body's inability to respond to and use available insulin.

Islet cell transplantation Transplanting the beta- (islet) cells from a donor pancreas and putting them into a person whose pancreas has stopped producing insulin. The beta-cells make the insulin that the body needs to use glucose for energy.

Islets of Langerhans Special groups of cells in the pancreas that secrete insulin.

Ketoacidosis See: Diabetic ketoacidosis.

Ketone bodies Chemicals produced by the body when body fat is broken down and used for energy.

Ketonuria Having ketone bodies in the urine; a warning sign of diabetic ketoacidosis (DKA).

Kidney disease Any one of several chronic conditions that are caused by damage to the cells of the kidney.

Kidneys Two organs in the lower back that clean waste and poisons from the blood.

Lancet A fine, sharp-pointed blade or needle for pricking the skin.

Laser therapy Using a special strong beam of light of one colour (laser) to heal a damaged area. A person with diabetes might be treated with a laser beam to heal blood vessels in the eye.

Lipid A term for fat.

Lipodystrophy Lumps or small dents in the skin that form when a person keeps injecting the needle in the same spot.

Macrovascular disease A disease of the large blood vessels that occurs when fat and blood clots build up in the large blood vessels and stick to the vessel walls.

Metabolism The term for the chemical changes in the body's cells that form the basis of life.

Microalbuminuria The presence of small amounts of albumin, a protein, in the urine. Microalbuminuria is an early sign of kidney damage.

Microaneurysm A small swelling that forms on the side of tiny blood vessels. These small swellings may break and bleed into nearby tissue. People with diabetes sometimes get microaneurysms in the retina of the eye.

Microvascular disease Disease of the smallest blood vessels caused by the walls of the vessels becoming weakened.

Myocardial infarction Also called a heart attack; results from permanent damage to an area of the heart muscle. This happens when the blood supply to the area is interrupted because of narrowed or blocked blood vessels.

Nephrologist A doctor who sees and treats people with kidney diseases.

Nephropathy Disease of the kidneys caused by damage to the small blood vessels or to the units in the kidneys that clean the blood.

Neurologist A doctor who sees and treats people with problems of the nervous system.

Neuropathy Disease of the nervous system.

Nutrition The process by which the body draws nutrients from food and uses them to make or mend its cells.

Nutritionist See: Dietitian.

Obesity A condition in which a greater than normal amount of fat is in the body; more severe than overweight; having a body mass index (BMI) of 30 or more.

Ophthalmologist A doctor who sees and treats people with eye problems or diseases.

Optometrist A person professionally trained to test the eyes and to detect and treat eye problems and some diseases by prescribing and adapting corrective lenses and other optical aids and by suggesting eye exercise programmes.

Oral glucose tolerance test (OGTT) A test to see if a person has diabetes. See: Glucose tolerance test.

Oral hypoglycaemic agents Pills or capsules that people take to lower the level of glucose in the blood.

Pancreas An organ behind the lower part of the stomach that is about the size of a hand. It makes insulin and enzymes that help the body digest food.

Pancreas transplant A surgical procedure that involves replacing the pancreas of a person who has diabetes with a healthy pancreas that can make insulin. The healthy pancreas comes from a donor who has just died or from a living relative. A person can donate half a pancreas and still live normally.

Peripheral neuropathy Nerve damage, usually affecting the feet and legs; causing pain, numbness or a tingling feeling.

Peripheral vascular disease (PVD) Disease in the large blood vessels of the arms, legs and feet.

Peritoneal dialysis A way to clean the blood of people who have kidney disease.

Pharmacist A person trained to dispense medicines and to give information about them.

Photocoagulation Using a special strong beam of light (laser) to seal off bleeding blood vessels such as in the eye. The laser can also burn away blood vessels that should not have grown in the eye. This is the main treatment for diabetic retinopathy.

Podiatrist A doctor who treats and takes care of people's feet.

Podiatry The care and treatment of human feet in health and disease.

Polydipsia Continuing thirst that is often a symptom of diabetes.

Polyphagia Continuing hunger that is often associated with weight loss and may be a symptom of diabetes.

Polyuria Producing large amounts of urine. Associated with polydipsia and often a symptom of diabetes.

Postprandial blood glucose Blood taken 1–2 hours after eating to test for the amount of glucose in the blood.

Prevalence The number of people in a given group or population who are reported to have a disease.

Proliferative retinopathy A disease of the small blood vessels of the retina of the eye.

Protein One of the three main classes of food. The body's cells need proteins to grow and to mend themselves. Protein is found in many foods such as meat, fish, poultry, and eggs.

Proteinuria Too much protein in the urine. This may be a sign of kidney damage.

Rebound A swing to a high level of glucose in the blood after having a low level.

Receptors Areas on the outer part of a cell that allow the cell to join or bind to insulin that is in the blood.

Renal A term that means having something to do with the kidneys.

Renal threshold The level at which the kidneys excrete substances from the blood to lower levels.

Retina The centre part of the back lining of the eye that senses light.

Retinopathy A disease of the small blood vessels in the retina of the eye.

Risk factor Anything that raises the chance that a person will get a disease.

Self-monitoring of blood glucose (SMBG) A way as person can test how much glucose is in the blood. Also called home blood glucose monitoring.

Stroke Disease caused by damage to blood vessels in the brain.

Subcutaneous injection Putting an injection just under the skin.

Symptom A sign of a disease.

Syndrome A set of signs or a series of events occurring together that make up a disease or health problem.

Syringe A device used to inject medications or other liquids into body tissues.

Systemic A word used to describe conditions that affect the entire body.

Triglyceride A type of blood fat.

Ulcer A break in the skin; a deep sore.

Unit of insulin The basic measure of insulin.

Urine testing Checking urine to see if it contains glucose and/or ketones. Special strips of paper or tablets (called reagents) are put into a small amount of urine or urine plus water. Changes in the colour of the strip show the amount of glucose or ketones in the urine.

Urologist A doctor who sees men and women for treatment of the urinary tract and men for treatment of the genital organs.

Vascular Relating to the body's blood vessels (arteries, veins, and capillaries).

Vitreous humor The clear jelly (gel) that fills the centre of the eye.

Index

Note: Page numbers in *italics* refer to illustrations

195